The Midwife and Society

Also by the same authors and from Macmillan

THE SOCIAL MEANING OF MIDWIFERY

The Midwife and Society

Perspectives, Policies and Practice

Anthea Symonds
Lecturer in Social Policy
University of Wales, Swansea

AND

Sheila C. Hunt
Professor of Midwifery
University of Central England and
Birmingham Women's Health Care NHS Trust

MACMILLAN

First published 1996 by
MACMILLAN PRESS LTD
Houndmills, Basingstoke, Hampshire RG21 6XS
and London
Companies and representatives
throughout the world

ISBN 0-333-63038-6

A catalogue record for this book is available
from the British Library.

This book is printed on paper suitable for recycling and
made from fully managed and sustained forest sources

10	9	8	7	6	5	4	3	2	1
05	04	03	02	01	00	99	98	97	96

Printed in Great Britain by
Antony Rowe Ltd
Chippenham, Wiltshire

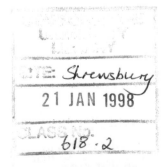

Dedicated to those midwives who are curious about the world
in which they live and are prepared to ask why

and

For my father, Joseph Eric Martin, who had a way with words

(Sheila C. Hunt)

Contents

viii · *Contents*

List of figures

List of tables

Foreword

Midwives are generally sceptical of politics, even with a small 'p', and have only slowly begun to realise that political naivety is both dangerous and diminishing. Anthea Symonds' and Sheila Hunt's excellent text will surely demonstrate to them that understanding the sociological context in which they practise midwifery is also a prerequisite for attaining that proper political perspective, without which the art and science of midwifery will not prosper or develop to meet the ever-changing needs of the public we all serve.

This book provides a thought-provoking look at our professional practice and identifies its many-faceted background, particularly in relation to power and its proper use, roles, gender and health inequalities.

Not all the observations are comfortable for us and the book challenges us to look anew at our stereotypes and unresearched practices. My hope is that all midwives will read this book and reflect upon their practice in the light of the empowerment it provides. In his *Essay on Human Understanding* the philosopher John Locke (1632–1704) said, 'It is one thing to show a man that he is in error and another to put him in possession of the truth.'

Anthea and Sheila put us in possession of some very important truths vital to the continuance of our present attempts to achieve a renaissance for midwifery. This book could be the grit in the oyster and stimulate midwives to develop creative practice of the highest standard. Truly a pearl beyond price!

SARAH ROCH

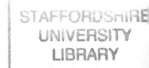

Acknowledgements

The authors and publishers acknowledge with thanks permission from the following to reproduce copyright material: Open University Press, for Table 2.6, from D. Pilgrim and A. Rogers, *A Sociology of Mental Health and Illness* (1993); NPEU, Radcliffe Infirmary, Oxford, for Figure 2.7, from A. Macfarlane *et al.*, *Counting the Changes in Childbirth: Trends and Gaps in National Statistics* (1995); Social Policy Association, for Table 5.1, from P. Selman, 'Teenage Motherhood Then and Now: comparison of the pattern and outcomes of teenage pregnancy in England and Wales in the 1960s and 1980s' (July 1994); *The Independent*, for Figure 6.2 (15 August 1995); Routledge, for Table 7.5, from R. Forrest and A. Murie, *Selling the Welfare State: The Privatisation of Public Housing* (1988).

List of abbreviations

AIMS   Association for the Improvement of Maternity Services
ALRA   Abortion Law Reform Association
ARM   Association of Radical Midwives
BMA   British Medical Association
CMB   Central Midwives Board
DoH   Department of Health
DOMINO   Domicilary In and Out (i.e. care by midwife at home, hospital admission for a brief period (6 hrs) only for the birth of baby, then post natal care at home)
EOC   Equal Opportunities Commission
ESRC   Economic and Social Research Council
GMC   General Medical Council
GP   general practitioner
HBA   households below average income
LIF   low-income families
MA   Maternity Allowances
MIDIRS   Midwives Information and Resource Service
MoH   Ministry of Health
NCT   National Childbirth Trust
OPCS   Office of Population Censuses and Surveys
RCM   Royal College of Midwives
RCN   Royal College of Nursing
RCOG   Royal College of Obstetricians and Gynaecologists
SMP   Statutory Maternity Pay
SPUC   Society for the Protection of the Unborn Child
UKCC   United Kingdom Central Council for Nursing, Midwifery and Health Visiting

Introduction

This book is essentially a guide to a general sociological perspective and to social policies which are significant both for midwives and for women and their families. It is not an introduction to either sociology or social policy but should be seen as a map which readers may use to guide them to further study, reading or thinking about some of the issues raised.

Midwives are a part of society not just as midwives but as women, wives, mothers, daughters, partners, tenants and consumers, and as such they are affected by social policies in their everyday lives. (Throughout this book midwives will be referred to as women as this is statistically and culturally the most accurate, men representing only 0.2 per cent of practising midwives [UKCC, 1994]). Likewise, the women for whom they care also play many roles, they are not just prospective mothers but may be workers and carers for others. Being pregnant is a very small but important segment of their lives: it is not the total of their lives.

In order to 'make sense' of the changing society in which they work, midwives will, we hope, find this book both interesting and challenging. It puts forward some ideas with which you may not agree. This is its purpose, to provoke analytical thought and discussion. It employs a 'woman-centred' approach – that is, it focuses upon female experiences and upon the effects of policies on women. It cannot tell the student everything there is to know in these fields and there are bound to be omissions. The book is offered as a starting-point and as a guide to making sense of the social world in which midwives practise. Some students will be fascinated by the insights and will decide to develop their interest in the topics further. Some will find that understanding some of the concepts will add a new dimension to their midwifery care and encourage them to think and question more.

The danger implicit in any book like this is to assume that the authors are writing for undergraduate sociology and social policy students or at least are preparing mini-sociologists and mini-scholars of social policy. This is not the aim. The book is aimed at midwives and students of midwifery undertaking Diploma (level 2) and Degree (level 3) studies. Even midwives undertaking Masters degrees may find the text helpful. It aims to enhance the preparation of the midwife or inform the continuing education of the qualified midwife, so that she becomes more analytical, more thoughtful, more responsive, more understanding and more able to offer women appropriate, sympathetic, sensitive and realistic advice. To do this, today's midwife must be informed, well-educated and articulate. To rely on common sense is inadequate as common sense is ill-informed and based only on experience. It would be a great shame if the real value of sociology and social policy study for midwives was misunderstood. Midwives work in society. Society constructs the environment, manufactures the issues, sets the policy and deals with the fall out. Midwives give the care in that environment, to ignore the wider context of care and the issues therein is to diminish the care women receive.

This book is divided into two parts. Part I, containing the first five chapters, focuses on sociological theory and its application to midwifery practice. The contents of these chapters are intertwined and the links with midwifery practice are like society itself, neither simple nor straight-forward. Many of the issues and concepts in this book do not exist in isolation but are interconnected. The questions and discussion points are linked to each chapter but information in other chapters will assist students in developing an understanding of the issues. At the end of Chapters 1, 2, 3, and 4 are case studies followed by questions and discussion points.

Part II, containing the remaining three chapters, is concerned with issues in social policy. Families, communities, women and midwives are considered and again the questions and discussion points draw on evidence in all chapters.

Chapter 1 gives an initial introduction into the academic discipline of sociology. It explains how sociology is a means of perceiving and theorising about the social world in which we live and suggests that when midwives study sociology and society in a more thoughtful and analytical way, they will begin to think more analytically about the care they give to women.

Chapter 2, on 'Social Divisions and Patterns of Inequality', is an especially important chapter and illustrates how sociologists attempt to explain divisions in society. It gives particular attention to social class, race, ethnicity, gender and age. This chapter offers definitions, suggests some causes of poverty, and considers some studies from the midwifery literature.

Chapter 3 offers sociological perspectives of the family and community and reveals that there is not just one model of the family but many different formations. The chapter explores not only ideologies of the family and community but also some of the myths and half-truths surrounding these concepts. The case studies in this chapter (as in the first two) are designed to help midwives to understand the different roles and responsibilities which women have in different households, so that they may offer appropriate care and advice to women and their partners.

Chapter 4 is called 'The Social Aspects of Pregnancy and Childbirth'. It explores birth as a social and cultural event and the domination and medicalisation of birth in a patriarchal culture.

Chapter 5 explores the myths of motherhood and describes how it has been socially defined, limited and constructed. It explores post-natal illness and concludes that it is not simply a physical illness with a physical cause. Theories on bonding are considered and the role of fathers in birth and beyond.

Chapter 6 is the opening chapter of Part II and deals with issues in social policies. This chapter encourages the reader to be aware of policies on state benefits, marriage, divorce, children, etc., but more importantly to consider why social policy has been framed in the way it has. The reader will consider which theories underpin decisions in social policy and why gender roles have been institutionalised into health and welfare systems in Britain. This chapter includes questions and discussion points designed to encourage midwives to apply theory to aspects of clinical midwifery practice.

Chapter 7 is also about social policy and it describes how theories of the male-breadwinner role have shaped social policies. This chapter focuses on women and considers such issues as abortion, maternity benefits, and child care. Policies on housing and homelessness are considered and again the questions and discussion points are related to aspects of midwifery practice.

Chapter 8 explores the nature of professionalism and its significance and application for midwifery. It explores the social aspects of a profession and considers the influence of social class, gender and ethnicity in a professional group. The statutory control of midwifery is discussed as is the new control of the professions, 'managerialism'.

The case studies in this book are based on real-life situations. Such is the nature of midwifery practice that sometimes real life is more surprising and stranger than fiction. All the names are fictitious.

This is a book for students and midwives who are able to make use of relevant knowledge from a range of sources, who can explain, summarise, develop logical clear arguments, make links between areas of work, be independent, imaginative, creative and critical. Midwives who use this book should become more thoughtful, more analytical, more sceptical, more responsive and more able to generate new ways of providing midwifery care. This is the aim of the text.

Sociological Theory Applied to Midwifery

Chapter 1

What is sociology?

Midwifery care takes place in many different environments, with many different types of people and many different groups. The midwife of the 1990s is concerned with the care and well-being of women and their families before conception, throughout pregnancy, childbirth and the post natal period. Her role is demanding. Her care must be responsive to the individual needs of women, proactive in anticipating needs, reactive to changing needs, and reflective in that she thoughtfully considers her care. She must consider if the care that was offered was appropriate, relevant and went some way towards meeting the needs of the woman and her family as they experienced the changes that childbirth brings. It is increasingly important that the midwife of today should understand the environment of care and something of the society where that care takes place.

Midwives study sociology in order to challenge assumptions, to become more analytical, and more questioning of the world around them. Sociology provides a framework for thinking about midwifery care in the context of that care. It enables the midwife to ask why, how, who, what if, and when.

This chapter is intended to give an initial introduction to the academic discipline of sociology. Obviously, this can be only a basic sketch but it is hoped that it will reveal its basic characteristics and objectives. Sociology is a means of perceiving and theorising about the social world in which we live. It is hoped that by studying society in this more analytical and thoughtful way midwives will enhance their work practice and that they, and the women for whom they care, will enhance their experience of birth.

Sociology as a specific intellectual discipline emerged in Europe against the background of turmoil and change which preceded and encompassed the French Revolution towards the end of the eighteenth century. This was a period in which all the old certainties and beliefs about the societal order were being challenged. This time became known as 'The Enlightenment' as it was characterised by a belief in science and rationality as opposed to the preceding eras of superstition and ignorance. Logical reasoning and a stress upon the experimental method of knowledge accumulation underpinned this new way of seeing the world.

The term 'sociology' (from Greek and meaning science of society) was first used by the philosopher, Auguste Comte. Comte believed that human societies could be studied and analysed in the same way as any other phenomena such as plants, animals and the movement of the planets. Sociology, for Comte, meant that scientific Laws on societal development and change could be constructed. In many ways this represented a search for order and understanding of human development in societies which appeared to be haphazard and mysterious. To a certain extent both these trends – the belief in analytical study and the search for a framework of understanding – still form the basis of much of sociology. Sociologists do not believe that 'things just happen', they search for an explanation for social action, the existence of institutions, belief systems, and inequalities between groups in a society. Peter and Brigitte Berger (1976) characterised the sociologist as the person who constantly asks 'Who says so?' Primarily, it challenges a belief in the 'naturalness' of the *social* world. Explanations for inequality or the power of societal institutions which are centred on a belief that certain forms of behaviour are 'natural' or 'inborn' are rejected by sociology. Instead sociologists look for the way in which society itself has constructed and perpetuated so-called 'natural' attributes.

Although, as we shall see, within sociology itself there are differing modes of explanation and schools of thought, all sociologists to a greater or lesser extent tackle the nature of the relationship between the individual and society. All human beings are unique in that no two people are physically or intellectually identical. Nevertheless, groups of people are held together by certain similar beliefs and threads of common experience and shared economic and social interests which enable us to analyse and construct theories about ways in which specific sets of individuals can be said to make up a definable grouping. Sociology could be termed a search for the understanding of the way in which a society works, a recognition that individual differences are subsumed within a network of group similarities and a constant questioning of beliefs and everyday realities. This perpetual questioning of taken-for-granted assumptions, beliefs and institutions makes sociology a fascinating but frequently 'uncomfortable' exercise.

■ **Understanding how society works**

In seeking to understand how a society develops and changes whilst maintaining continuity, sociologists focus upon two main components; social *processes* and social *structures*. Social processes are the mechanisms by which individuals learn the social 'rules' of their surrounding society. The description of a 'process' in this context is akin to that used in industrial production. The raw material (new-born human) is subjected to many agencies and influences which mould and construct them into the desired finished product – a conforming member of society who 'fits' into his/her place.

One of the most important of all social processes is socialisation. This is the mechanism by which, first the family, and then other agencies within society, like the education system, religious and political beliefs, and the surrounding culture and value system teach the individual the appropriate patterns of acting and thinking. People learn to become social beings within the prescribed limits of their society and historical time. In this way a person gains a sense of identity, of gender, social class, ethnicity and nationality. They learn to 'fit in' with their surrounding group culture.

This does not necessarily mean, however, that this is a completely closed system. People are not totally the product of their socialisation but often 'negotiate' with what they are being taught. If this did not happen society and society's beliefs and behaviour patterns would never change. Socialisation is an ongoing and dynamic process in constant movement. For example, children in the earlier part of this century were viewed as undeveloped adults with few social rights and were subjected to strict control and discipline. The socialisation of nearly all children was based upon this premise: they were constructed as subordinate to adults in every way. But today children are seen as individuals with their own specific needs and demands and with legislative rights. The way in which many children are socialised into being assertive and having a central place in a family system and in legislation was almost unthinkable a couple of generations ago. As society's ideas and needs change so does the content of the 'message' communicated but the actual process of socialisation is always continuing. This is not to put forward the view that people are totally programmed into conformity, for as we shall see, there are many divergent views within sociology on the relationship between the individual and society. Many other aspects of life are viewed as social processes – marriage, work, childbirth, ageing – and the important emphasis is on the aspect of the social, for all these experiences are placed within the cultural value system of a particular society at a specific time. Marriage and childbirth in the British culture has different meanings for different groups within British society at any one time and can, of course, change over time. This is what sociologists mean by a 'social meaning' of an activity like childbirth or an occupation like midwifery: they are processes through which people gain their own social identity but which must be placed within the context of the surrounding society.

This surrounding society is composed of social structures. These are seemingly solid and static institutions in which individuals live out their lives. They often appear remote and abstract and having an autonomous existence separate from the individuals within them. The family is one such structure for we often refer to 'the family' as an institution which often seems to exist as a separate entity with a life of its own. Politicians talk of 'family values' and legislation is enacted with 'the family' as a focus. Social structures like the family, the economy, the legal system, education system, and religion affect the way in which individuals live their lives but at the same time they are also constructed by human societies. Social structures too are subject to change and they have a history of their own.

Sociologists analyse the composition and purpose of these structures, they ask questions like: How do they work? What are the aims and objectives? Who has power within them? Social processes and social structures have so far been presented as separate from each other but often a particular social phenomenon will be used by sociologists as both a process and a structure at the same time. For instance, gender could be said to be both a process and a structure. Children are socialised into the appropriate and expected belief and behaviour systems for their gender identity. This message is carried by all the socialisation agencies in different forms from advertising images to medical science textbooks. But at the same time, gender identities do not carry equal power, for despite changes over time, to be a female in British society is still to be placed in a relatively subordinate position. This is why many feminist writers would argue that gender acts as a structure in that it determines both the way in which people have unequal access to economic power as well as a process of personal identification. In this way, gender can be a seemingly solid structure as well as a fluid social process. Social class, race, age and deviance are also often described as both processes and structures. In searching for an understanding of the way in which a society actually works, the role of ideas and beliefs is of central importance.

■ Where do ideas and beliefs come from ?

The study of the dominating *culture* of a society which overarches all processes and structures is central to a sociological understanding. The sociological definition of a culture is a very wide one involving beliefs, ideas, behaviour patterns, and traditions. A culture also includes aspects of everyday life including food, clothes, jokes, games, all of which need to be sociologically understood and explained.

How is a culture created and what purpose does it serve ? The first step in answering this question is to make the point that cultures are diverse, they differ between countries and nations and over time as well as differing within the same society at the same time. But there also exists a dominant set of ideas and beliefs in any society at any one specific historical period, which sets the agenda for the workings of social processes and structures and reflects the power structure of a society. Many different groups within a society will have their own cultures or sets of beliefs and behaviour patterns: there are youth cultures, class cultures, ethnic cultures and occupational cultures. An occupational culture such as that which operates within midwifery or nursing is one which includes working practices, beliefs and attitudes, codes of language and dress and ways of joking and communicating which define the nature of that occupational identity. Newcomers are socialised (process) into the 'rules' of the culture and learn to 'fit in' to the system (structure) but this culture exists within, and to a certain extent reflects, the dominant societal culture.

Cultures, then, give a sense of belonging and identity but can also be oppositional in some way to the dominant one. For instance a drug culture involves all the aspects of any other sub-culture, but is seen as 'deviant' to the mainstream value system.

Learning to belong to a culture is a social process, but the culture itself takes on the aspect of a social structure.

This view of a culture as both a structure and a process is one which will be used in this book particularly to look at the way in which the dominant culture constructs ideas of motherhood.

A culture is the structure within which an individual gains a sense of place. It gives an anchorage of gender, social class and ethnic belonging. The transmission of a culture is a process too: it is the means by which a person 'makes sense 'of the world around them. But it is important to remember that for a sociological analysis, any culture is essentially a *social construction*. No set of ideas about the world is a natural or ageless phenomenon, all ideas have a *social and historical* root. This includes scientific theories, political philosophies, religious beliefs and everyday 'facts' and behaviour patterns. Sociology as an academic discipline too has its social and historical roots, sociological theories and models of society have changed and been redefined throughout the past two centuries.

■ Sociology and theory

Sociology then is not a static body of knowledge but a dynamic one which is constantly alert and alive to changes in societies and in new ways of analysing these changes. New schools of thought and ways of analysis have arisen and been applied to an understanding of society. A theory is an attempt to make sense of the causation and consequence of social change, it is a set of connecting beliefs on *why* certain things have occurred in the way they have and also to posit some prediction of the future. If one asks the question why? in reference to any event then almost certainly one will be faced with a set of differing and perhaps oppositional replies. This is also true of sociology, in answer to the questions of why certain processes and structures have developed in the way they have and what the relationship is between an individual and her/his society, different theoretical perspectives have constructed alternative answers. This is the nature of the sociological practice – it is a discursive and constantly questioning discipline.

Traditionally there have been three main schools of thought or theoretical disciplines in sociology, which stemmed from three theorists, who were often known as the Founding Fathers (traditional sociology was not immune from gendered language). Generations of sociology students were introduced to the perspectives of Marx, Weber and Durkheim in this way and several libraries of books exist on the works of these three thinkers (McLellan, 1979; Giddens, 1971; Jones, 1986). In recent years these perspectives have been enlarged and incorporated into new perspectives such as feminism, structuralism, post-structuralism and post-modernism. As if this were not enough, the basic disciplines themselves have fragmented and so there are Marxisms not just Marxism, feminisms not one feminism, and neo-Weberianism as well as functionalism and structural functionalism.

For people who are attempting to work as full-time midwives and not full-time sociologists this array must appear overwhelming, and impossible to gain an understanding of any of them. But sociologists would find the biological and physiological theories of childbirth just as bewildering !

What all these theories have in common is that they are attempting to answer the question why and how societies are constructed the way they are. If we take one concept – that of power in society – and through that trace the differing perspectives then perhaps we can gain a basic understanding of their divergent theories.

■ Sociological theories of power

All sociological theories accept that power relations exist. All societies have had structures and hierarchies of power. Sociological theories approach the study of power in two ways: first, they seek to identify these groups in society which have power, the basis of this and how it is used, and, second, the nature of the power and the way in which it is transmitted and reproduced in society.

■ Marxism(s)

Marxism as a means of analysis is not an homogeneous approach. There are at least two distinct schools within Marxism which give a different emphasis on aspects of power: Classical Marxism and Neo-Marxism. *Classical Marxism* otherwise known as economic determinism, or functionalist/mechanistic Marxism, is the view purveyed in *Das Kapital* and the *Communist Manifesto* which attributed the basis of power in any society to the economic base. This base is defined as what is produced in an economy, how and by whom, how it is exchanged and who owns the means of production and exchange. Within this economic base relations of production are created between those who own (bourgeoisie) and those whose labour produces the goods (proletariat). This is essentially an unequal relationship, as the profit to the owners is accrued out of the exploitation of the labour time of the workers. In short, those who labour do not receive their full entitlement as a profit has to be made within a capitalist economic system. The relationship between these two classes is essentially one of perpetual conflict of interest and struggle for power. The ruling class gain further economic power and this is transmitted to all other structures of society. Thus the power of the ruling class is reinforced by the legal system, it is transmitted via the agencies of the family, the education system, religion and the whole cultural milieu. This power permeates and creates a dominant ideology which seeks to subsume everybody within it. Thus all of society is organised in the interests of this one group but it is represented as being in the universal interest. 'The ruling ideas of every epoch are those of the ruling class' (Marx and Engels, 1970). In this view, the basis of all power is economic and the culture or ideology which is constructed by the powerful ruling class only seeks to convince the powerless of the just and 'natural' aspect of their own inferior position. This is a structural view of power, in that it is vast objective economic structures which determine individual beliefs and actions rather than the conscious actions of individuals or groups.

This emphasis in Marxist thought on the determining nature of the economic base was redefined in the 1960s by Marxist writers and thinkers who became known as *Neo-Marxists*. This brand of Marxism is often described as voluntaristic or humanist and sought to move away from the stress on economic determinism and look at the role of culture and ideology within people's life practices and beliefs. Based very much on the work of the Italian Marxist writer, Antonio Gramsci (1971), who died in a Fascist prison in 1940, this strand of Marxist analysis has had a great impact on many current European theorists. Gramsci perceived capitalist society as being successful in reproducing an ideology of dominant ideas which he argued had gained *hegemony* and constructed a whole way of experiencing and understanding the world.

This term has become much-used in sociology. It refers to the position of overarching power gained by an idea at a particular historical time. For instance, ideas of the market as the most efficient way of producing and exchanging goods and services gained hegemony in Britain during the 1980s. This does not mean that everyone in Britain agreed with this view, but it was through this belief that all political and public debates were conducted.

Gramsci therefore laid as great a stress on the role of ideology and culture as on the economic. He believed that capitalist society was not just divided into two main antagonistic classes but into many fragmented class factions which came together at certain times to form alliances around and within certain sets of ideas. In this view, ideas themselves do not 'naturally' belong to any one class but can be appropriated by different class formations and alliances. When one set of ideas gains hegemony, the class alliances formed within this set of ideas also gains a position of hegemonic power. For example, ideas on the necessity of the welfare state in the early post-war period in Britain gained hegemony and were represented by groups such as the professional middle class, organised labour, women's groups and some factions of the capitalist class especially those in manufacturing. This interpretation of power looks at the power of groups to set political agendas within which all discussion and conflict takes place. Gramsci, like Weber, stressed the importance of *legitimation* by ruling groups by means of control over the actual subjects which are debated and by setting the parameters within which all alternative discussions are placed. Take, for example, the belief that 'the family' is a good institution which must be defended. This means that all debates on how to support the family may differ on actual means but the basic premise will be accepted by all. This Marxist approach then stresses the importance of a study of popular culture and cultural apparatuses (the mass media) and the different ways in which a message can be interpreted by individuals. Although it does not reject the importance of the economic in the construction of power it seeks to understand how this power is transmitted and reproduced via ideology and culture.

A Marxist analysis then stresses above all the conflict which is inherent in society based upon unequal power in the economic relations of production and reproduced in powerful ideologies.

■ Functionalism and power

Functionalism is the broad label given to those who see society as an interconnection of interdependent parts all of which have a function in maintaining the continuity of society as a whole. Emile Durkheim is regarded as the most influential of the functionalist theorists. Writing at a time when France was undergoing great social and economic upheaval at the end of the nineteenth century, he was concerned to look at how societies could hold together and construct a social cement which would integrate different groups and create a collective conscience. As Marxists emphasise conflict, so functionalists emphasise an essential consensus operating within societies. Critics of this approach often say that within this emphasis on cohesion and integration, there is no concept of power relations. It is the interdependence of occupations and groups which is stressed. Durkheim (1964) looked at the division of labour in modern industrial societies as essentially one of linked need and function.

But later functionalist sociologists especially those of the American school such as Talcot Parsons (Parsons 1954) and Davis and Moore (1945) emphasised the just and functional nature of unequal rewards in society. Parsons stressed the legitimate use of authority by social institutions as a means of organising for the good of all the society. In this view, certain occupations were more functional and required a longer period of training which required a sacrifice from students. Thus it was only just that these positions of power should be more highly rewarded later on. In this way not only was social stratification seen as functional and legitimate but also it was recognised that the positions of high social status should be open to those of merit and talent who were willing to undergo early sacrifices. This is a vision of a more 'open' society with acquired status as the ideal rather than a system of ascribed privilege.

All functionalist thinkers from Durkheim onwards have emphasised the importance of a cultural system which integrates individuals into the dominant values of society. Conformity to the norms and beliefs of society is essential and Parsons argued, basically a 'natural' desire. Socialisation agencies such as the family, school, religion and mass media all work to produce this level of desired conformity which is in the interests of all as everyone gains a reward even if these are not of equal value. It is the integration and cohesion of society itself which is of the utmost importance.

Both Marxist and functionalist theorists viewed society as somehow 'outside' the individual. It is societal structures and social forces which act upon individuals and which makes every individual act an essentially *social* one. For Marxists this included the social construction of ideas and beliefs and for Durkheim it included the seemingly individualistic act of suicide. The third approach of the 'Founders', that of Weber and action theory took a different approach.

■ Weber, belief systems and power

Weber took as his main object of study the meaning that people give their actions within a given society. All human actions are meaningful he argued : whether they are *normative*, that is, actions which conform to the norms of a society and are not given any real thought by the participants, or *purposive*, that is, actions which are deliberately engaged upon to produce certain objectives.

For Weber, the belief system of a society was its core dynamic, and only by *understanding* (*verstehen*) this could actions be truly understood. Most of his work (Weber, 1930) in this respect concerned the religious belief systems of different societies and how these guided the meaning placed upon human action. He argued that the religious belief system of Calvinist Protestantism which emerged in Northern Europe in the seventeenth century signalled a change in the meaning placed upon economic and social activity. The emphasis on the value of thrift and hard work which he labelled 'the Protestant Ethic' set the ideological framework for the values of the capitalist enterprise.

Weber (1948) was also concerned to analyse the dimensions of power and authority. He distinguished between these two concepts in that power could be overt and based upon violent oppression which elicited normative obedience from the population and was based upon coercion, and authority which was perceived as legitimate by the population and elicited a purposive response. For example, if held at knife-point most people would obey an attacker's commands without accepting the legitimacy of this, but a government may demand money in the form of taxes and most people, although they may resent it, would nevertheless obey because they recognise its legitimate right to do so. The imposition of the 'poll tax' was a good example of this: it was a deeply unpopular measure but most people paid because of the legitimate authority of government. All power seeks to become legitimate authority. Weber then analysed certain patterns of authority from the traditional authority of the patriarch, to the charismatic authority of the demagogue, and the legal–rational system of authority which was personified by democratic and bureaucratic modern states. This concept of legitimation of authority has been taken up by many Marxists who have studied the ways in which this process has taken place in societies.

Unlike Marx however, Weber did not see power as the property of one economic class but he viewed power as present in three main spheres:

- party (the power of political groups).
- class (defined in a much more varied way to include occupational rewards and access to market services and consumer goods)
- status (the degree of prestige which specific positions have in society).

These three spheres are obviously connected in that those who wield political power often come from a specific class background and acquire status, but this is not always the case. It is not only those who were born into the ruling class who achieve political power and status. Power therefore may be acquired and people have varying degrees of life-chances in the gaining of power and status. Weber's model of society is less rigid than that of either Marx or Durkheim.

Weber's theoretical approach with its emphasis on the importance of understanding individual action within a society influenced a school of analysis known as *interactionism*.

■ Labelling and roles

This became very influential in America in the 1960s and concentrated upon an understanding of the social interaction between groups of individuals. It was much used in studies of deviance and tended to place an equal value upon the belief system of both the 'deviant' and mainstream society. The two writers most associated with this view are Howard Becker (1973) and Erving Goffman (1961a, 1961b). It was from these approaches within the phenomenological perspective that *labelling theory* evolved. This was the theoretical view which identified deviant behaviour as that which had been so labelled, and asked the question, which behaviour and which groups of individuals become labelled as deviants and by whom?

Goffman's work is of special interest to health-care professionals as he studied the institutionalisation of human behaviour especially in mental hospitals (Goffman, 1961a). He argued that once given the label of 'mentally ill', a person's subsequent life and actions were interpreted by others within the light of that definition. Once the label has been applied even the most ordinary action would be seen as that of a mentally disturbed person thus producing a stigmatised condition.

This approach signalled a move away from a sociological view of society as existing 'out there' to be studied in a scientific and objective way and a recognition that society was itself created and constantly reinforcing its values and norms through everyday actions. Goffman (1961a) argued that a person's identity was one which that person themselves had constructed and then presented to others. This is a 'dramaturgical' view of society, where people play roles as in the theatre. So that the way you dress, talk, even move is the 'presentation' you make to the outside world which is the audience. Sociology of course, as well as drama, uses the idea of a *role*.

Structural functionalist sociologists too were very taken with the idea of people learning to conform to set roles within a society which reinforced the norms and values of that society. Parsons (1964), for example, wrote of the way in which people conform to a 'sick role' when ill.

In a sense the personal sphere of life within which social processes operated became as important an area of study as societal structures. It was the belief that the 'personal is political' and that people are socialised into performing certain roles in society especially those which identified people as masculine or feminine that feminist thought articulated. A gender identity like other identities, was learned behaviour and not an expression of inborn 'natural' characteristics: this was the argument which feminist writers were to take up.

■ Feminism(s)

By the beginning of the 1960s a feminist perspective on accepted values and beliefs began to be popularly and academically expressed. Betty Friedan (1963) put into words the 'problem with no name', a discontent felt by many women especially in the affluent economies of America and Europe about the limitations placed upon their role as housewives and mothers. This manifested into a theoretical approach which sought to place the female experience of the social world in the centre of sociological analysis.

Sociology, in this respect had been as male-dominated as any other discipline, as Ann Oakley (1974b) argued, with its concentration on male occupations, male school experiences and male deviancy and youth cultures. Social class was defined by the male occupation for the purpose of social surveys and the stratification system was one in which women became 'invisible'(see also Chapter 7). In Britain, the first sociological studies of women's lives appeared at this time (Gavron, 1966; Oakley, 1974a, 1974b). Feminism was to have a great impact on many branches of academic study: in history, for example, many studies of the lives of women which had been largely ignored by most male historians emerged. Sheila Rowbotham (1973) argued that women had been 'hidden from history', and a mass of work evolved which sought to give a female presence to much of the previously male-based accounts.

There was not, however, a unified and homogeneous feminist analysis. As with Marxism, within a feminist theoretical approach there existed differing emphases and models of power. What they all had in common however was a broad agreement on the existence of a *patriarchal system* as the dominant structure in society. Power and authority it was argued, belonged both to the male culture and to individual males in social structures, and in everyday life that was the broad basis of the approach. A feminist approach sought to analyse the reasons for this masculinist power position and its continuance, its function to a capitalist mode of production, its legitimation, and the internalisation by both men and women of its 'naturalness'. Given this wide range of areas of study as well as attempts to pose an alternative way of interpreting the social world, a unified feminist approach inevitably became fragmented into different schools of thought. Some writers laid stress on the social process of learning gender roles. The early socialisation of children, especially of girls, into the appropriate beliefs and behaviour patterns through differential treatment by parents (especially mothers) and the use of gender-appropriate toys and books was one area of study (Oakley, 1985).

Other studies looked at the role of gender in education and the way in which girls and boys were separated into studying gender-appropriate subjects with the result that girls 'learned to lose'. The pervading power of language in reproducing and legitimising male domination was also the focus of feminist study (Spender, 1990; Lees, 1986). Within this analysis not only was it demonstrated that words themselves constructed a male view of the world for example, chair*man*, the *man* in the street, *man*kind, but also men themselves occupied a dominant position in the use of speech and language. Interestingly, even now in a predominantly female occupation such as midwifery or nursing the staffing levels are referred to as *man*power.

The use of sexual insults against women were also studied, the fact that they can be insulted for heterosexual activity, with words such as 'slag', 'scrubber', 'nympho', for which there is no masculine equivalent. Insults against male sexual activity only involved so-called deviant behaviour such as homosexuality. In other words, women were insulted for so-called 'normal' behaviour which in a man would be a source of compliments whereas men could only be insulted by referring to so-called 'deviant' sexuality.

Studies in schools (Spender, 1988) revealed that boys were allowed by teachers (both male and female) to interrupt more, to talk more loudly and demanded and were given more attention. Men by virtue of deeper and louder voices were also more acceptable in the realm of public speaking. Other studies took a more *structural* approach and looked at the economic position of women and their relatively powerless position in the workforce. Studies on domestic labour and its function to a capitalist economy became the Marxist–feminist focus of interest (Delphy, 1984). As we shall see in Chapter 3, the role of women in studies of 'the family' was a great contribution to an analysis of the social system.

Motherhood and the control of female sexuality was a dominating concern of much feminist scholarship in both sociology and psychology. One of the most powerful and controversial arguments came from Shulamith Firestone (1970) when she expounded a 'radical feminist' view that the task of feminism was to 'free women from their biology' and use technologies of artificial reproduction. This was opposed by another wing of feminist writing which saw motherhood as an 'essential' part of a female experience but one which had been appropriated by the male medical establishment (Oakley, 1984; Kitzinger, 1978, 1980a, 1980b). Other writers took up this theme and feminist histories of the marginalisation of female midwifery became set reading for many professional courses (Donnison, 1977; Chamberlain, 1981). Another emphasis of feminist writing was to look at motherhood and child-rearing as a *socially constructed* role for women and focused upon the social and economic inequality which women as mothers suffered (Riley, 1984; Wilson, 1977).

In recent years there has been widespread criticism of much feminist scholarship from black and Asian women who have argued that the overwhelming focus has been upon the experiences of white women. Black women, it is argued suffer a 'double jeopardy' and discrimination.

A feminist approach although many-faceted and with differing political and philosophical beliefs, sees power and authority in social structures in the domain of males and a masculine-based culture.

■ Foucault, post-modernism and discourses of power

The social theories of post-modernism or post-Fordism have in the past decade become new ways of analysing modern industrial societies. As the phrase 'post-modern' suggests, this view is based upon the belief that modern industrial societies have moved to another stage of development, from large homogeneous structures to fragmentation into smaller units. The sort of industrial production and organisation of large factories and assembly line working which characterised the late nineteenth and most of the twentieth centuries is said to have been replaced by smaller units, self-employment and 'cottage' industries. The production of Ford motor cars in America at the end of the last century was the first process to use assembly-line methods. Because this type of production was so fast and efficient in turning out vast numbers of standard models using unskilled but reasonably well-paid labour on the production line, this whole method of working became known as Fordist. The description of post-Fordism is now applied to all large organisations which have moved away from this model and are now engaged in splitting up production into smaller units. The reorganisation of the Health Service with its emphasis on dividing purchasing and providing and using outside agencies has been described as 'being in a stage of post-Fordism'.

Within this school of social thought, much attention is paid to the values of *consumption* rather than production and to the diverse nature of cultural and belief systems and social processes and structures.

This approach denies the totality of a class- or (male-) based power structure and looks instead to the ways in which a 'social meaning' is placed upon certain structures and processes in society. This is an essentially fluid and ever-changing perspective on power which sees power as being present in many aspects of everyday life and not belonging exclusively to any one group or class.

One of the many theorists who have argued that societies are to be understood in terms of their diversity of power through social and political discourses, was Michel Foucault (1980a, 1980b). His work is of special importance to health-care professionals as he was concerned to place a scientific or medical discourse as a powerful influence in the social construction of 'the truth' in modern societies. By tracing the history of the treatment of the insane (Foucault, 1973) in Europe from the Middle Ages, he articulated the theory that the main problem for modernising and industrialising states was the control of the newly mobile and increasing population. The means by which this population could be controlled and organised was found within the creation of the prison system, hospitals and the 'medicalisation' of society. The mass had to be under the constant surveillance by the few. The design of prisons and later of hospitals, was to enable the perpetual observation of the controlled by the controllers. If you think of the Nightingale design of a hospital ward it is the perfect example of the Foucault argument about the power of spaces. The arrangement of the beds meant that many patients could be surveyed and controlled by just one nurse from a central nurses' station. This control was to be further extended so that the mass of people actually began to control themselves through the belief that they were being constantly watched and their every movement observed. This control extended to human bodies and they were literally 'opened up' to the scientific gaze with the advance of studies of anatomy. We will return to this argument in Chapter 4 when we discuss the social aspects of the use of ultra-scanning in pregnancy.

Other writers such as Donzelot have seen the creation by the state of 'social agents' like health visitors, doctors and social workers whose task it was to 'police' the family in the stage of developing industrialisation (Donzelot, 1970).

Foucault sees a system of beliefs and 'facts' which he terms 'discourses' as the means by which a society produces 'the truth' which is internalised by people in diverse ways and in differing degrees. But there is not one centre of power in these competing discourses, power is diffused throughout the social system and is present in social interaction, personal relationships and the use of language, and is legitimised by the discourse of the truth. This truth is historically specific: what is 'true' for one epoch will not be so for another. Nothing is static, nothing is solid, everything is in a dynamic relationship of constant change.

■ **Midwifery and sociology**

Why then should midwives both as students and in continuing midwifery education be encouraged to study sociology? After all midwifery is essentially a very practical activity where the main aim is to produce a live and healthy baby and a woman who is not damaged mentally or physically by the experience of childbirth. Studying sociology is likely to assist midwives in thinking beyond the immediate day-to-day demands of their profession.

Sociology as a discipline requires skills in analysis and synthesis. It is these skills that will eventually help the midwife to be more under-standing, think more about the care she offers and communicate more effectively with women. For many years many midwives have been taught to accept the norm and not to challenge assumptions. This culture of acceptance, subservience, and domination by medical men is explored elsewhere (Hunt and Symonds, 1995). Research evidence as a basis for midwifery practice has changed the way in which midwifery education is planned and offered. Students are taught to review the published literature and develop the ability to distinguish strong evidence from weak as well as to appreciate the physical, emotional and psychological effects of the care they offer.

There are many areas of midwifery practice, its rituals and routines, that are now being questioned and reviewed. Many of the old and established ways of delivering care have been rejected and previous assumptions are being reconsidered. Child bearing women are being helped to return to the place where they belong, which is at the centre of the maternity services. Reports such as *Changing Childbirth* (DOH, 1993) challenge midwives to listen to women and think more carefully about the how, the where and the when of the care they offer.

There is of course, a danger that in the new world new assumptions will merely replace the old ones. Studying and thinking about sociology may help midwives to be curious about the world in which they live, work and offer care to women, and enable them to ask the right questions. It is hoped that this questioning, thinking and challenging will lead them to think before accepting new rituals and routines.

For example, the themes of choice, control and continuity of carer explored in *Changing Childbirth* could so easily become mere rhetoric. But continuity of carer improves the quality of communication between women and midwives. When communication is good, women are more likely to feel in control of the childbirth experience and more able to understand the implications of the choices that are available to them.

This chapter has introduced midwives to some sociological theories and challenges them to consider in more detail the societal processes and the structures that form the backdrop to the maternity services in the 1990s and to ask themselves these questions , 'Where is midwifery now?' and 'What has led to this, the British way of birth?' It is hoped that midwives reading this book will think, perpetually challenge and refuse to accept the norm, as only then is childbirth likely to become a better experience for women and for families.

In the following case studies, which are based on real life events and which draw on material from all chapters in the book, you are asked to think about the social processes and structures in which maternity care takes place. The aim is to offer a focus for discussion and to help the reader to apply some complex theories from other disciplines to the practice of midwifery. In real life some things happen that cannot be slotted into neat chapters of a book. In the same way, in each case study there is some overlap and use of material from other chapters.

┌─ **Case Study 1.1** ──────────────────────────────────────┐

This is the story of a fictitious ordinary family and their first encounter with the maternity services. The couple's names are John and Sue. They are not married but have lived together in what could be described as a 'stable relationship' for seven years. John has been employed as a manual worker since he left school but is now unemployed. Sue was previously married but is now divorced. She works part-time, some weeks full-time, as a factory worker. Her work involves fitting microchips to handsets of portable television sets. She enjoys the company of other women and she considers herself well-paid, especially on the weeks where she has lots of overtime. She intends to return to work as soon as possible after the birth of her child. She describes herself as 'the main wage earner'. John seems to flinch as she describes herself in this way but he comments that there is very little work about.

This is Sue's second pregnancy, her first ended in a termination when she was 16 years old. This followed a 'one-night stand' at a party when she was drunk. She explains that she drinks 'a lot', mainly cider and smokes around 10 cigarettes a day. She is now 23 and John is 24 years old. They seem to be happy in each other's company but state that 'they don't like hospitals much'. At the start of the booking interview, Sue asks tentatively if she will be free to go to work for the afternoon shift. She says she is sorry to cause 'a fuss'.

They bought their council house in 1989 but they are now in arrears with the mortgage. The house is in need of repair, the roof leaks and the central heating system is broken. The house is now worth less than the £35000 they paid for it. They say that it is a constant source of worry but they also believe they will not be evicted if a baby is on the way. John says that he wishes Sue had not persuaded him to buy the house. He said that he believed that the social security would have looked after them if they had a child. The couple used to be entitled to housing benefit, but this stopped when Sue's income rose beyond the threshold for payment.

Both parents appear to be delighted about the pregnancy and talk excitedly about the birth. The place of birth is assumed to be the hospital. John explains early in conversation that he would like a son and that he has already bought a Manchester United top and a small pair of football boots.

└──┘

■ Questions and discussion points

- How can studying sociology and social policy help this midwife in understanding this family and their needs?
- What does the case history tell us about the changing role of the family and marriage?
- Who might hold the power during this interview?
- Do you believe that the midwife has legitimate power? If the answer is 'yes' on what basis can she use that power? (Consider aspects of power, knowledge and authority.)
- Does the site of the booking interview affect the power balance?
- What does the case history tell us about the changing roles of men and women?

- What does the case history tell us about the beliefs, values and cultural norms of this couple?
- How will an understanding of social stratification (class) help the midwife offer appropriate care?
- Is the social class of this couple likely to affect the outcome of pregnancy? How might the pregnancy be affected?
- What are the inherent risks of the couple's life style?
- Would it make any difference to the balance of power in this encounter if the midwife was black and from a working-class family?
- How would you describe the social construction or the meaning of pregnancy in this case study?

Most of the answers to these questions are within the chapters of this book. John and Sue are a couple living in today's society. They are a changing family and subject to changes in social policies. The midwife is better placed to offer good care when she understands more of the complexities of the world in which John and Sue have a baby.

Key points

Sociology
- is a means of thinking, perceiving, understanding and theorising about the world in which we live.
- is a systematic study of human society that provides evidence and explanations of how society works.
- is a means of offering explanations and evidence of action of individuals and groups.
- attempts to explain the distribution of power, social resources, economic and political power.
- is concerned with individuals operating in a social world and with trying to understand how the 'social world' works by investigating social structures and social processes.
- investigates how social structures and relationships develop, persist and change.
- is a specific intellectual discipline that emerged in Europe against a background of turmoil and change – the French Revolution.
- is a discipline where old certainties are challenged.
- is a search for order – it assumes things do not just happen; sociologists search for explanations.
- asks what is the relationship between individuals and the society in which they find themselves.
- is a questioning of all 'taken for granted' assumptions.
- it seeks to understand how society works.

Sociologists are concerned with issues such as :
- Power – subordination/ exclusion/ inclusion
- Systems and sub-systems
- Institutions
- Roles
- Norms
- Gender – sexual divisions of labour
- Social construction of caring
- Feminism (s)
- Families and welfare state
- Socialisation, health
- Communities
- Care in the community
- Personal responsibility
- Social stratification
- Social class
- Inequalities in health
- Class and health – social class, gradients in health
- Poverty in the welfare state
- Relative and absolute poverty
- Politics of poverty
- Ethnicity and race
- Race and health
- Equal opportunities
- Disability
- Health beliefs

Chapter 2

Social divisions and patterns of inequality

In the course of their work, midwives will meet the rich and the poor and will observe how all types of people adapt to the major life changes associated with pregnancy and childbirth. Sociologists offer explanations and some keys to understanding inequality, poverty and deprivation. Such explanations can help midwives to understand the context of care, to accept in a non-judgemental way individuals' life-styles, and enable them to offer appropriate care to all women and their families.

The main focus of sociological study and theories is the description and explanation of social divisions and inequalities which exist in all societies. All sociologists have proffered some analysis of these divisions, and looked for patterns of inequalities which would explain why certain *groups* of people experience relative deprivation in society. What are the characteristics which deprived groups have in common?

If we concentrate on just British society as an example of a modern industrial state in the late twentieth century we can detect certain patterns to group inequalities. As we shall see, Britain as a whole shares some similar characteristics with other European countries and with the USA, and it also differs from other societies. Within Britain too, there are great differences between areas, regions and within the population, so there are geographical as well as social divisions.

Sociologists, it must be remembered, are not intent on offering explanations for an individual's relative success or failure but seek to look for group patterns. The fact that one person rises from poverty to become a self-made millionaire is often celebrated simply because it is the *exception* in all societies rather than the rule. Sociologists are interested in explaining why the majority of people do not achieve a much higher status and position of power than the one into which they were born, and not why the exceptional individual does. Sociological explanations of divisions, are based upon what different perspectives show to be the main factors of stratification. These factors are social class, race or ethnicity, gender and age. These are in the nature of initial labels or classifications and form the beginning of a wider analysis. Social scientists need first to identify groups so that they can calculate the actual types and extent of relative deprivation and inequality. This is a categorisation of groups not individuals. We can always identify the odd individual who does not 'fit' into any strict category, but this is not the point. In order to get an overall view of divisions and inequalities in modern British society we must first clearly set out the factors by which we are identifying people.

The next step is to define what we mean by inequality. We are all unequal to others in some respects: some are taller, slimmer, stronger, can run faster or have the ability to learn languages, but these are not patterns of inequality, they are individual differences spread throughout the population (although this spread is not random). When does 'difference' become 'inequality' ? In order to address this question we return to the concept of power which was discussed in the previous chapter. This includes the power to gain money and consumer goods, to obtain access to services such as education, housing and health. This power of course, is not distributed equally. What degree of power over their social and working lives do different groups possess? From the moment a baby is born, his/her access to a certain standard of living, to good health and even to a longer life span is influenced by the baby's social identity. Therefore in order to trace these patterns it is essential that we construct a means by which groups can be identified and then we can begin a comparative analysis. Traditionally sociological analysis centred upon occupational and economic characteristics as being all-important, but as we shall see, sociologists now refer to other social divisions as being equally crucial.

■ Social class

The concept of class is one which dominates sociology and social research. Many people argue that it also dominates English (rather than British) society and culture! In sociology the label of class is used in two different ways; first, it is a classification which is used in social research, in government census, and in market research and opinion polling; second, it is a concept which underpins all theoretical debates on the causes and explanations of differentials in power.

□ Measuring class differences

The use of the classification for social research began in 1911 in order to investigate the variations in the death rates of the population. In 1921, it was structured on a basis of the skill (not earnings) which was required to do certain jobs, and was based upon the occupation of the *male* 'head of household'. This has remained broadly in place until the present day. The definition of high or low skill was, of course, a subjective one, and resulted in all non-manual jobs being regarded as needing more skill than manual ones. It also relegated women to a secondary status judged upon their

Table 2.1 Registrar-General's classification of social class

Social class		Examples of occupations
I	Professional	Lawyer, doctor,
II	Intermediate	Teacher, midwife, manager
III	N/M skilled non-manual	Clerical, shop assistant
III	M skilled manual	Electrician, mechanic
IV	Semi-skilled manual	Farm worker, fitter
V	Unskilled manual	Cleaner, assembly-line operator

husband's, or if unmarried, their father's occupation which was often statistically inaccurate as well as discriminatory. There was also no place for housewives, unemployed or retired people – it was purely an occupational scale. Nevertheless, this is the Registrar-General's system of classification as shown in Table 2.1. Despite its inadequacies, this model did, to some extent, reflect the occupational structure of British society throughout most of the inter- and post-war years. But in the past decade this structure has changed almost beyond recognition. The growth in self-employment, part-time working, women's employment, redundancy and 'early' retirement and unemployment, as well as the change in the type of jobs, with the decline in skilled manual jobs and the increase in the service and information industries have rendered this model practically obsolete. This was officially recognised in 1995, when the Office of Population Censuses and Surveys (OPCS) commissioned a study to update the classification system. It was estimated by the Economic and Social Research Council in the subsequent report that as many as 40 per cent of the population was excluded from official classification and that this group probably included the most disadvantaged in society. Therefore, social and medical research as well as the allocation of government funding for a whole range of social welfare provision including housing grants and cash for health authorities, would be based upon a totally inaccurate identification of the population. The OPCS are also considering the construction of a new system altogether which could measure the amount of power people have to control their own lives; this would include household incomes, educational qualifications, and possessions. These wider categories have already been used in health research to study indices of deprivation. But it should be remembered that a change in the classification system will mean that comparisons of data will be difficult to make over time.

The most widely used indicator is the Jarman scale (Jarman, 1983,1984). This was used by Townsend in the Bristol study (Townsend *et al.*, 1985) in an attempt to measure areas of deprivation for resource allocation purposes. The Jarman scale attempts to score under-privileged areas on indices such as:

- children aged under 5;
- numbers of ethnic minorities, and single-parent households;
- elderly living alone;
- overcrowding;
- poor housing;
- numbers of non-married couples;
- low social classes.

This enables researchers to identify specific clusters of deprivation rather than individual groups of people. The Department of the Environment also adopted a similar scheme for identifying areas of deprivation. This methodology does produce some anomalies, Margaret Whitehead (1988) reported that in both the Jarman scale and the one used by the Department of the Environment, London emerged as possessing the majority of 'most-deprived' areas with none being found in the North of England – a finding which contradicts observation and all other evidence. The reason for this anomaly was the existence in many London boroughs of a relatively high percentage of ethnic minorities and single mothers which had the statistical effect of 'skewing' the results. But despite some inadequacies, these and other methods (Whitehead, 1988) do represent an attempt to overcome the inappropriate nature of the occupational scale and to identify areas of need and deprivation. But areas or clusters of people sharing the same housing and standards of living will of course be influenced by social class, gender, ethnicity, age, disability and other factors. The area index is therefore a picture of the concentration of social divisions in one area. This is another feature of modern British society, the fragmentation of areas. In Victorian urban and rural areas there existed a strict separation of rich and poor but now there is a far greater 'mixing' of wealth and poverty in the same approximate location. We will return to the geographical element in patterns of inequality later in this chapter.

This classification of occupational class has been one of the tools of the trade for social research for most of this century. But the concept of class is a very complex one which many sociologists have addressed in differing ways.

☐ The meaning of class

Marx was the first to define and theorise the meaning of class in a capitalist society. As we saw from Chapter 1, he posited a basic two-class model, composed of the bourgeoisie who owned the means of production and the proletariat who sold their labour power, so that the class position of a person was determined by his/her role in production, and this was an objective category set by economic factors. But for Marx, class was also a cultural or ideological category. People occupying the same position in

the production process shared a consciousness of class, he argued. This meant that the working-class perceived that they had interests in common and that these were opposed to those of the ruling class. Eventually, this class-consciousness would result in a revolution in which the workers would overthrow the system which kept them in a position of exploitation. But this concept of consciousness has proved a difficult and complex one for subsequent Marxist writers and theorists.

The increasing complexity and fragmentation of occupations and ownership in modern industrial capitalist societies have rendered this basic two-class model very difficult for observers to apply. It could be argued that in the nineteenth century, a person's social class was immediately obvious, the wealthy bourgeoisie were well-fed and expensively dressed, and occupied a totally separate world from that of the impoverished working-class. The middle- and upper classes were physically very different in that they were, on average, much taller and weighed more than the lower classes. This difference is apparent even in films of the 1940s and 1950s where working-class people were seen variously as figures of fun, cowards, slow but kind, but above all, deferential.

By the 1960s however, with the advent of universal education, health care provision, state welfare benefits and housing as well as a mass consumer market it was often argued that class differences had become eradicated. The economic boom of the period with its emphasis on youth cultures made it possible for many young working-class people to become successful, working-class wages rose in real terms and these factors led some sociologists to talk of the 'end of ideology' (Bell, 1960) and of class divisions.

So does the concept of social class still have a meaning for sociologists? In fact the 1980s and 1990s have seen an increased interest in the classification and analysis of class divisions. During the 1980s, the expansion of many financial businesses, especially in the City of London, and the subsequent growth in consumerism created a 'new' social grouping, the Yuppies. As in the 1960s, this social grouping was composed of young people who gained money and status through new markets, this time those of the Stock Exchange and the boom in property. At the same time and almost as a mirror-image of the 'new wealthy' there arose a description of the 'new poor' in British society. This group was and still is characterised by its marginal position both geographically and socially. The homeless sleeping in cardboard boxes in public thoroughfares, beggars on the streets of most large cities, the riots on bleak out-of-town housing estates and in the inner cities, all contribute to a definition of a social group unseen since the Victorian age. This group appears to exist outside mainstream society and is seen as a threat to the existing social fabric.

This perceived fragmentation of British society into the 'have lots', the 'haves' and the 'have nots' cut across traditional sociological definitions of social class. Britain experienced a period of rapid social and economic change and disruption during the 1980s, which is still continuing, and these changes rendered many of the definitions of social class either inappropriate or obsolete. The greatest impact of economic change was felt by both the older heavy industries and manufacturing, sectors which had been the base of employment for the traditional working class in modern times. This meant that whole areas which had been formed around a single occupation or industry such as mines, shipyards or steelworks were irrevocably changed when these industries closed down. In a relatively short space of time, ways of life which had been constructed by male employment and classified by sociologists as typifying a 'working-class' identity, practically disappeared. Many commentators argued that this fragmentation of social life was a part of the process of post-modernism (see Chapter 1), but it raised problems for the sociological analysis of social class. Sociology in a sense is still grappling with this problem of analysing modern Britain in terms of social class composition. This is, of course, why the Registrar-General's Classification has been changed. The advent of an 'under-class' in British society has become one of the most controversial debates within British and American sociology (Murray, 1990; Mann, 1992; Morris, 1994). But much of the description of this group centres on its culture or belief system, the so-called 'dependency culture', rather than just focusing upon its economic position. The analysis of social class by reference to the class possession of belief systems within which ways of living are constructed has long been an important part of a sociological approach.

☐ Class cultures

The definition of a homogeneous working-class culture was often rejected by sociologists who tended to view divisions within the working class as being of great significance. The distinction between the 'respectable' and the 'rough', for example, was one of the most significant (Carter, 1966; Hoggart, 1955). Although the working class has always been fragmented by regional, ethnic and occupational differences (Bourke, 1994), this process accelerated in the 1960s.

Studies (Goldthorpe and Lockwood, 1968; Lockwood, 1989) described the emergence of a new type of culture unlike that of the traditional working-class and based upon a more 'privatised' life-style. This, it was said, was indicative of the new generation of workers who placed the possession of consumer goods and individual achievement above collective interests. Within a traditional working-class culture, it was argued, there was a belief in collective action and a loyalty to organisations such as trade unions which illustrated this commitment. Another strong attitude was that of fatalism, an acceptance of the part that luck and fate played in one's fortunes. This was often accompanied by a hedonism which resulted from this belief that the future could not be planned for or perceived ('You could get run over by a bus tomorrow') and so instant pleasure was seen as a sensible measure.

A traditional middle-class culture, on the other hand, was based upon 'deferred gratification' – that is, the willingness to do without in the present in the belief that this would pay dividends in the future. The trappings of a middle-class life-style were based upon this belief. Children were encouraged to stay on at school to gain qualifications rather than leave early to get a paid but 'dead-end' job. The hardship involved in buying a house on a mortgage, the career structure of many professional occupations which meant that you began at the bottom and worked your way to the top in later years were all acceptable. This concept even pervaded marriage and conception: the age at which middle-class couples married and had children was, on average much later than the working-class. Sociologists conducted studies on many areas of class cultural differences, especially in the explanations of working-class 'failure' in education which was put down to parental attitudes, the different language codes of the classes (Bernstein, 1977), the cultural bias of the curriculum itself (Young, 1971). All these were studied in great depth.

Class cultures, it was argued (Willis, 1980; Hall and Jefferson, 1975), allowed people to make sense of the world around them, a world over which groups within the working class had less power of control than had members of the middle-classes. A class-based culture could be seen as a means by which less-powerful groups were dominated by others, or the way in which they negotiated within the system for a larger space for themselves, or as a means of resistance (Parkin, 1971). Some sociologists interpreted increasing vandalism (Cohen and Taylor, 1992), clashes between different youth groups (Hall and Jefferson, 1975) as means of resistance to oppression. This way of analysing class cultures is still basically a Marxist one, with its recognition of class exploitation and the demands of a capitalist economy for the social division of labour. These cultures were seen as the product of the economic and social system.

But how do we perceive social class differences on a day-to-day basis? What 'messages' of class identity are picked up and interpreted by observers ? Clothes, speech, body language, even the type of car we drive and the music to which we listen are influenced by a perception by ourselves and others of social class or status. This image and self-identity of class is very pervasive and requires a conscious effort to alter in order to fit in with another class group. The way in which the hairdresser in the film *Educating Rita* slowly altered her appearance, tastes and even the way she walked, so that she could 'pass' as a middle-class student was a brilliant illustration of this presentation. But this is not to adopt a purely 'dramaturgical' view of the world as posed by Goffman (see Chapter 1), for social class is not just a matter of appearances, these are effects but not causes of class as a social division.

But what does this mean for midwives and midwifery care? Changes in appearance are effects of social division but they also have the power to affect the relationship between the woman and the midwife and the quality of care. When a woman walks into an antenatal clinic or a hospital labour ward she is still often meeting a stranger. The midwife, makes a quick assessment, often informed by information in the maternity record, and taking her cues from external appearances decides on her style of care. This places a woman at an extraordinary disadvantage. Assumptions are made and care delivered on the basis of appearances. Whilst midwives traditionally have the skill to form a relationship with a woman very quickly, the midwife would be well advised to check out her assumptions and care with the woman concerned. To 'assume' can make an 'Ass' out of 'u' and 'me'!

Is social class then ultimately about the possession of money and therefore, power? A definition which was based more upon status than class identity as defined by ownership of the means of production (Marx) was put forward by Weber. He saw class as being made up of many components based upon financial rewards, working conditions, employment prospects, consumer power and the political influence which could be utilised: all these factors added to what he called one's 'life-chances'. In many ways, this is an easier definition for most people to relate to on an everyday basis. But there are certain national cultural differences to be considered when applying this definition of status. British society is perhaps more 'closed' to new wealth and social mobility than American society. There still exists a rejection of outsiders even if they possess money. The institutions of British economic life like the City and the Stock Exchange have become more open in recent years but is there still a hidden level of entrenched traditional power there? But power structures exist not only in financial institutions, they are everywhere – in hospitals, schools, benefit offices – everywhere where there is social interaction. Social class can be defined as one of the processes by which these structures are maintained. As well as an indefinable but unmistakable image of class belonging which those of us socialised within the British culture recognise, there also exists another group of 'outsiders' within modern British society.

■ 'Race' and ethnicity

Sociologists tend to operate with a concept of 'ethnicity' rather than 'race'. Race tends to be a biological description whilst ethnicity denotes a cultural identity. Like social class, ethnicity is applied in two ways in sociology – as a measuring tool in social research and as an explanation for patterns of inequality.

Since the early nineteenth century, Britain has become an increasingly multicultural and multiethnic society, although of course the very definition of Britishness itself is multifaceted culturally as it includes not only the English, but the Scots, Welsh and Irish as well as smaller groupings like the Cornish and Manx.

In the early nineteenth century the Irish settled in England and Scotland in particularly large numbers when they came to work in the large construction projects, notably the building of the canals and railways, which were the foundations of industrialisation. Irish communities can be found in most large urban areas with London, Liverpool and Glasgow being the areas of biggest population settlement.

Jewish immigration into Britain occurred in the late nineteenth century, and stemmed largely from Eastern Europe where they were victims of vicious pogroms. By far the greatest percentage of Jewish immigrants went to America (as did the Irish after the famine of 1846), but there were Jewish settlements in the East End of London, Manchester and Leeds, by the beginning of the twentieth century. The Jews, unlike the Irish, did not become a part of the British industrial proletariat but brought with them trades and skills which previously did not exist in British society. Most notable among these were the methods of mass production in the garment industry and different retailing techniques. The advent of cheaper fashionable clothes produced for a mass market and the creation of a 'one price' stall which eventually led to the Marks and Spencer empire are illustrations of this unique contribution to British economic and social life.

Throughout the 1930s and after the war, European immigration into Britain grew. This was mainly from areas of eastern Europe which were then within the Soviet Union, but also from Italy, Greece, Malta and Cyprus (the two last-mentioned were previously part of the British Empire). After the Communist victory in China in 1948, Chinese migration from Hong Kong which was (until 1997) a British protectorate also increased. All these groups contributed in many ways to new directions in British economic and social life, including of course, restaurants, clothes and food shops, and hairdressers.

However, it was in the 1950s that the phrase 'immigrant' took on a new and coded meaning for the word 'black'. Many West Indian men had served in the British forces during the war and sought to remain in Britain afterwards. They were joined by the first immigrants from the West Indies who arrived in 1953 and settled in London and other large urban areas. The expansion in the National Health Service and transport especially meant that there were job vacancies in these areas of the newly formed welfare state and it was to the former colonies that Britain looked for recruits.

Table 2.2 Ethnic group composition of the population, 1992, per cent

Region	WHITE	ETH. MIN.	BLACK	B–C	B–A	B–O	SOUTH AS	IND	PAK	BAN	CHIN/O	CHIN	O–AS	O–O	TOTAL POPULATION (000)
Great Britain	94.5	5.5	1.6	0.9	0.4	0.3	2.7	1.5	0.9	0.3	1.2	0.3	0.4	0.5	54 888.8
England & Wales	94.1	5.9	1.8	1.0	0.4	0.4	2.9	1.7	0.9	0.3	1.2	0.3	0.4	0.6	49 890.3
England	93.8	6.2	1.9	1.1	0.4	0.4	3.0	1.8	1.0	0.3	1.3	0.3	0.4	0.6	47 055.2
Wales	98.5	1.5	0.3	0.1	0.1	0.1	0.6	0.2	0.2	0.1	0.6	0.2	0.1	0.3	2 835.1
Scotland	98.7	1.3	0.1	0.0	0.1	0.1	0.6	0.2	0.4	0.0	0.5	0.2	0.1	0.2	4 998.6

Source: Adapted from Owen (1992).

Note: all percentages are rounded up.

B–C	Black–Caribbean
B–A	Black–African
B–O	Black–other
SOUTH AS	South Asian
IND	Indian
PAK	Pakistan
BAN	Bangladesh
CHIN/O	Chinese and others
CHIN	Chinese
O–AS	Other Asian
O–O	Other–Other

By the 1960s, immigration from the Caribbean had been augmented from other former colonies, from Asia and especially from India. The areas of settlement were those in the East and West Midlands, London, and other urban areas especially those where the textile and heavy industries were recruiting workers as well as the growing state sector, notably the health service. This is the historical background to immigration into Britain What must be remembered is that by the 1990s, it is no longer accurate to talk of 'immigrants' as now over 50 per cent of people of ethnic minority origin in the UK have been born here. Ethnicity, has now become, like social class, a way of identifying social trends, population changes and inequalities. Table 2.2 shows the ethnic group composition of the population.

It is important to note that for purposes of calculation, these classifications are far from adequate. There is only one category for the 'white' population whereas the ethnic population is widely gradated. For social research this means that we cannot accurately calculate divisions or inequalities *within* the 'white' population and so certain groups who may be relatively disadvantaged remain hidden. How ethnicity is defined is another grey area, what of people of mixed race?

The significant demographic difference between the ethnic groups however is one of age (Table 2.3). Ethnic minorities contain many more young people, and far fewer elderly pensioners.

Another significant factor about ethnic minorities is that the population is not widely or evenly dispersed but concentrated in certain areas, most of which had provided work and employment for the first generation of immigrants. In the past decade many of the industries in these areas have been hit by recession and unemployment and this has led to an exacerbation of areas of poverty and deprivation. An example of this is textile manufacturing. A recent study in Rochdale shows that the industry there employed a high proportion of Asian men and in 1971 over 16000 workers in total were employed in textiles; this had fallen to just over 3000 by 1984 (Penn, Martin, Scattergood, 1990) thus strengthening the link between ethnicity and unemployment. This has been termed the 'Americanisation' of British cities with, on the one hand, the close proximity of wealth and poverty and on the other, the formation of ghettos where all the social problems of deprivation are centred. Some members of ethnic minority groups have become over-represented in such areas. As Colin Brown has written, 'The position of black citizens of Britain largely remains, geographically and economically, that allocated to them as immigrant workers in the 1950s and 1960s' (Brown, 1988, p. 69). So how can we sociologically understand and explain this persistence of racial and ethnic inequality ?

A broadly Marxist approach would be to locate ethnic divisions within the overall class structure and define ethnicity as another form of class exploitation and conflict (Gabriel and Ben Tovim, 1978). Most members

Table 2.3 Population, Great Britain, by age and ethnic group, 1989–91

Ethnic group / Age group (%)	WI/G	IND	PAK	BAN	CHIN	AFR	ARAB	MIXED	OTH	ALL E M	WHITE	NS	ALLEG*
0–15	24	29	44	46	25	31	23	54	27	34	19	36	20
16–29	30	25	23	26	28	28	30	24	27	26	21	22	22
30–44	19	25	20	15	29	28	33	13	31	22	21	16	21
45–59	19	14	11	11	13	10	9	6	10	13	17	11	17
60+	9	6	3	3	5	2	5	3	4	5	21	15	20
All ages (= 100%) (thousands)	456	793	486	127	137	150	67	310	155	2 682	51 805	496	54 983

Note: *Including white and NS.
Sources: Adapted from *Labour Force Survey*; *Social Trends*, 23 (1993).

WI/G	West Indian or Guyanese	AFR	African	
IND	Indian	OTH	Other	
PAK	Pakistani	ALL E M	All ethnic minority groups	
BAN	Bangladeshi	NS	Non-specific	
CHIN	Chinese	ALL EG	All ethnic groups	

of ethnic minorities belong to the proletariat and therefore share with the white working class the same social relations of exploitation. But as Castles and Kosack (1973) wrote of the position of unskilled immigrant workers, they have short-term interests which may not coincide with the long-term ones of the indigenous working-class. So a Marxist analysis of racism would locate it firmly within the economic base and relations of production. But ethnicity and race are divisions over and above class. Not all ethnic minorities are in working-class occupations, but they are still likely to suffer from discrimination and disadvantage within a broadly middle-class and professional sphere.

We must also be careful not to use the term 'ethnic minority' in a generalised sense: there are probably greater divisions within minority groups. For instance, Indians are more represented among those with managerial and professional occupations than are those from the West Indian (Afro-Caribbean) or Guyanese, Pakistani or Bangladeshi populations. We have of course no way of differentiating between 'white' ethnic groups, so we cannot indicate proportion of Irish, Jewish, Welsh, Italian or Greek in any group of the population (see Table 2.4).

The other point to note is that for men, ethnic divisions in employment are more significant than for women. All women, regardless of ethnic origins, are more likely to be found in non-manual and clerical occupations, most of which are low paid and part-time. As with social class, theories of inequality often focus upon differing cultures and the stereotyping of minority groups by powerful majority groups. This process of 'labelling' often pervades education, health services, mass media and popular culture. Essential and 'innate differences' are often said to exist between ethnic groups. Within the British culture these stereotypes are familiar: 'West Indians are lazy but good-natured and excel at sport', 'Jews are sharp with money', 'the Irish are "stupid"', 'Asians are not to be trusted and are "unrealistically" ambitious'. These beliefs can then become entrenched and adopted in official organisations such as housing allocation, and so education, employment and 'life-chances' are affected by this institutionalised racism. We will discuss later on some of the ways in which these attitudes have pervaded the health service especially in relation to midwives' perceptions of the needs of Asian women.

The majority group has the power to label the minority and so right from the outset, some ethnic groups were defined as the providers of cheap labour or as a separate labour market from the 'white' majority. But this pattern also applied (perhaps to a lesser extent) to the Irish and the Jews as well as other groups, such as the Welsh and Italians.

The Weberian notion of status groups has also been used to analyse inequality and racism, and because this model supposes more fragmented class groupings, has been used often in sociology (Rex and Tomlinson, 1979). Status is seen as a separate but interlinked concept from class. But as Weber himself recognised, status and style of life are greatly dependent

Table 2.4 Employment, by broad occupation, ethnic origin and sex; average, Spring 1989–91; persons in employment aged 16 and over, Great Britain, per cent

Occupation	WHITE	EMG	WI/G	IND	PAK/BAN	ALL OTH
Men						
All non-manual	48	49	32	59	40	64
Managerial & professional	36	36	20	43	28	48
Clerical & related	5	6	*	9	*	8
Other non-manual	6	7	*	6	*	7
All manual	52	51	68	41	59	36
Crafts & similar	25	24	28	16	17	12
General labourers	1	1	*	*	*	*
Other manual	26	26	39	24	41	24
Women						
All non-manual	68	68	63	62	64	72
Managerial & professional	29	31	33	28	*	35
Clerical & related	30	29	26	27	*	30
Other non-manual	10	9	*	*	*	*
All manual	31	31	37	38	36	28
Crafts & similar	4	4	*	11	*	*
General labourers	0	*	*	*	*	*
Other manual	28	27	33	27	*	25

Note: *Including white and NS.

Sources: Adapted from House of Commons *Hansard* (21 May 1992).

EMG	Ethnic minority groups	PAK/BAN	Pakistani/Bangladeshi
WI/G	West Indian/Guyanese	ALL OTH	All other origins
IND	Indian		* Sample too small

upon economic power which is linked with social class. Status groups will therefore always bear a resemblance to social class and occupational membership but be defined by other factors as well.

Some groups possess a higher status than others within the 'host' society and culture, for example in the USA, the Irish as a group possess a higher status and greater political and economic power than they do in Britain. The question of status accruing to certain groups is an important one, for if the status is low then any occupation or area of housing occupied by such a group will itself become of a perceived lower and stigmatised status. People of the dominant culture then talk of neighbourhoods which 'have gone down' or jobs which 'used to be good'; the underlying code within such perceptions is that the presence of an 'outgroup' has adversely affected the previous higher status when occupied only by their own group. 'Outgroups' do not necessarily occupy a low status within a 'host' society, the history of British colonialism is evidence of that! The British occupation of India and areas of Africa for two centuries meant that it was the British culture and ethnicity which had high status and the surrounding majority 'host' culture was given a low status. The definition of status itself is then culturally determined and defined by social and economic power relations. A sociological analysis would concentrate therefore on explaining why certain groups had the power to label and discriminate against others and reject any belief in innate and inborn superiority or inferiority. This denial of the 'naturalness' of social divisions and inequality is most marked when analysing gender divisions in society.

We have said earlier that majority groups have the power to label minorities. There is evidence in the literature that midwives label women from ethnic minority groups and offer inappropriate care based on prejudice and racism. Bowler (1993) describes some findings from her 1990 study of Asian women and their experience of the maternity services. Using an ethnographic approach she found that midwives commonly used stereotypes to help them provide care. Midwives fell into the trap of assuming that all Asian women were 'difficult' and based their practice upon what the stereotypes led them to believe was appropriate care. They were inclined to accept a view of Asian women as a uniform or homogeneous group and thus characterised them as 'non-compliant', 'making a fuss about nothing' and lacking in normal maternal instinct. One midwife felt that she needed a one-page summary of all that she needed to know about Asians as she did not have time to read books!

■ Defining sex and gender

The most important point about the analysis of sex and gender is the definition of the two terms within sociology and social policy:

Sex denotes the biological status of male or female and is therefore used in classifications for social research.

Gender is of the greatest interest to sociologists as it is a concept which defines the cultural identity of men and women; their 'masculine' or 'feminine' characteristics, behaviour, appearance, beliefs and values.

As with social class, people present themselves as either 'masculine' or 'feminine' by means of codes of dress, speech, tastes, interests, which conform to society's expectations. The ways in which children learn their appropriate gender roles are discussed in more detail in following chapters, but it is important to note that for sociology, gender is seen as a social construction. The debate over 'nature' or 'nurture' is one which has dominated discussion on the roles of men and women for many years, as these are opposing explanations of difference and inequality.

In social research sex is used as a variable by which to measure inequality or as a means of defining and identifying social trends. In 1995, a detailed statistical portrait of women in Britain (HMSO, 1995) was published which gave a vivid picture of the lives of modern women and showed many aspects of lingering inequalities as well as improvements. The report revealed that over 12 million women, which is just over half of all women in the population, now undertake paid work, but only just over a quarter of these work in full-time jobs. However, in both manual and non-manual occupations women earn less than men and in 1994, 33 per cent of women received less than £200 per week compared with only 13 per cent of men (see Figure 2.1).

On the other hand, women now make up over 50 per cent of medical students and there are currently more female than male solicitors under the age of 30. However, women represented less than 5 per cent of High Court judges and less than 4 per cent of Appeal judges. In education, women make up 81 per cent of all nursery and primary teachers but only 57 per cent of head teachers, whilst in secondary education they represent 49 per cent of all teachers but only 30 per cent of heads.

The percentage of males on the UKCC (United Kingdom Central

Figure 2.1 Average gross weekly earnings, by gender, April 1994

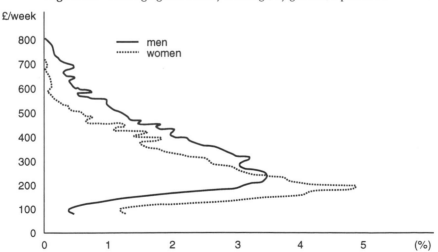

Sources: Adapted from OPCS (1994) and Central Statistics Office, *Social Focus on Women* (HMSO, 1995); reproduced in *Guardian* (9 August1995).

Council for Nursing, Midwifery and Health Visiting) effective register has risen steadily from 8.34 per cent in 1988 to 8.87 per cent in 1994. On Part 10 of the register (Registered Midwives) 99.8 per cent (35287) are female and 0.2 per cent (72) are male. Men however are well-represented in senior posts in management and in education.

The vast majority of women therefore work for less pay, and are not to be found in the upper echelons of political or economic power, despite great changes in recent years, Margaret Thatcher remains the exception not the norm!

We have already seen that the classification of occupational class renders women 'invisible' and this is one of the inadequacies of this classification as a tool of social research. But where women do appear as the focus of social research it is nearly always in their role within the family. Figures on birth rates, conceptions and abortions, contain only those for women, there are for instance, no statistics available on the numbers of fathers, married or unmarried!

The connection between women and responsibility for children is paramount in most research studies of poverty and homelessness and in indices of deprivation. It is as single mothers or lone pensioners that women are included in area deprivation indexes, not as women constituting a separate social group.

How can we explain the persistence of inequalities in life-chances for women? In many ways women have become more 'successful' than men in certain areas of social life. In education for example, girls gain more qualifications than boys even in subjects such as maths in which traditionally they failed. In subjects such as languages girls dominate, they are quicker in learning to communicate and are more 'advanced' at almost every level of childhood development. Women live longer; female babies and children have lower mortality rates and it could be said that they represent the 'stronger' sex.

Despite these advantages, women are more likely to be living in poverty both as mothers and in later life; they earn less than men throughout their working lives although they are more likely to be employed; they receive fewer benefits such as private medical insurance or private pensions, and as we have seen they do not reach positions of public or cultural power in our society. How can sociology explain this phenomenon?

■ Gender and patriarchal power

As we saw in the previous chapter, recent feminist approaches to this subject have looked at both the structure of inequality and the process by which female experiences are marginalised. In order to theorise this view fully the concept of *patriarchy* has been utilised. This refers to the dominance of masculine culture, values and power in societies although its original meaning is that of the rule of the father.

The division of modern society into 'public' and 'private' spheres (Davidoff and Hall, 1987) is very important to consider in this explanation. The 'public' sphere of the economy, politics and work became separated from the 'private' sphere of home, children and family with the onset of industrialisation, although as Davidoff and Hall have argued, the public and private spheres have never been truly separated and male power dominates both spheres. The public sphere which was dominated by men, however, became the defining one: all activities in the 'private' sphere which were undertaken by women were given a lower and marginalised status. Commentators have seen this division as a crucial one with the 'culture' of modern societies being defined as a male preserve as opposed to 'nature' which was female (Ortner, 1981). Simone de Beauvoir (1972) further argued that male experiences, history and interests thus became the 'norm' with female experiences becoming defined as 'Other'. This was especially true of the scientific culture which characterised modern industrial development. It can be illustrated in medical history when at the initial development of the study of anatomy it was only male bodies which were dissected and female bodies became seen as a 'mystery' and as 'abnormal' (Moscucci, 1990).

Writers such as Marina Warner (1976) have also argued that religious beliefs represent a masculinised value system with the person of God as a man and the role of women seen as that of 'mother' (the Virgin Mary) or 'whore' (Mary Magdalene) or household drudge (Martha). The worship of powerful goddesses is relegated to a primeval and pagan past (Stone, 1979). After all, it was only in 1994 that women were admitted into the Church of England as vicars and they are still not accepted as priests in the Roman Catholic Church or Greek and Russian Orthodox churches. The Hindu and Moslem faiths do not allow any measure of institutional power to women.

Males and females are culturally designated to distinct areas of activities and 'feminine' and 'masculine' pursuits and skills are defined not on their own worth but on the gender of the person performing them (Cockburn, 1990). This definition of skill as a gendered concept is one which has been used to explain the lower status of all female jobs and professions compared with male-dominated ones; the classic case is the disparity between both nursing and midwifery and the medical profession (we will discuss this further in Chapter 8). Medicine is a good example of both a male-dominated structure (women not admitted at all until the end of the nineteenth century) and an ideology (women are too emotional to make scientific diagnosis). Even though there are now equal numbers of women and men training in medical schools, the career prospects for women in medicine remain relatively poor (see Chapter 8).

Jeff Hearn (1992) powerfully argues that there is not just one form of

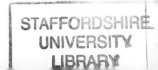

such patriarchal power but many patriarchies. He puts forward the definition of a public patriarchy which, since the nineteenth century, has come to dominate all public institutions, working life and the private female-based sphere of the home. Public patriarchy is seen in the increased role of the State in family life via state agencies of social work, health visiting and other forms of control. Even though some of the agents were themselves women, the control they exercised was over other women within this male-based power. This public patriarchy swept aside private patriarchy, so that the state and institutions such as education and social services actually took the place of the father of the family and rendered him superfluous. But women and children remain within the sphere of public male power even if the father is 'absent'.

The power to define and 'label' belongs to the powerful social groups, and men as a group have the economic and social power both to define and restrict women's behaviour. Women may complain of male behaviour and criticise men among themselves, but as a group they do not possess the power to define or control men. This does not apply to *all* men but as a group possession, masculine-based power operates very obviously in the public arena. Men as a group 'belong' in the public world of the street, work, pubs, in a way in which women and some other men do not. A good example of this can be seen in the case of attacks on women in a certain area which are always accompanied by the police and the media issuing warnings to women not to go out alone at night, but the obvious solution of ordering a curfew on men unaccompanied by a woman wandering the streets remains in the realm of the unthinkable!

It must be remembered that patriarchy is rule of the father, and fathers rule over sons and other men as well as women and girls. Hearn makes the point that class, ethnicity, age and sexuality all cross over in the exercise of patriarchal power, so that middle-class men control working-class men, white men control black men, middle-aged men control young and old men, the non-disabled control the disabled, and heterosexuals control homosexuals. The so-called 'public' world of the street and open spaces such as parks and school playgrounds, can be dangerous for certain groups of males as well as females.

A sociological analysis of the roots of cultural power can reveal how widespread and deeply pervasive ideas of 'masculine' and 'feminine' rights and duties have become. But when attempts are made to analyse the causes of inequality, it must be remembered that social class, ethnicity and gender and age constantly criss-cross each other.

■ Age

Anthropological studies of pre-industrial tribal societies show that they also have patterns of stratification and inequalities and these have been bascd upon age sets, with the greater power accruing to the elders of the tribe. Age, in many of these societies is of a high status and confers privileges. Many people argue that in Western societies the opposite is now the case and that age is one of the greatest factors of inequality. Sociological analyses of ageing follow two paths:

1. The pinpointing of age as one of the most important group charac-teristics in explanations of structured economic and social inequality (Phillipson, 1982)
2. The definition of an ideology which defined older people in certain ways, that of ageism (Bytheway, 1995).

Interestingly, the concept of a fixed retirement age is a recent one and the age varies between countries. Within the EU the official retirement age stretches from 60 for both men and women in France and Belgium to 67 in Denmark. In Britain, it was set at 60 for women and 65 for men under the Beveridge proposals enacted in 1945, although this has recently been altered to 65 for both (to come into effect in 2010). This setting of an age limit to full economic activity has meant that age has become one of the variables by which income, poverty rates, family status and health are measured. Figure 2.2 illustrates the composition of the older section of the population.

However, definitions of age have both a structural and sociological significance. Older people, especially older women, who are in the majority of older people living alone, are more vulnerable to poverty. An ageing population also has significance for decisions on resource allocation for the health service, housing and benefits.

Figure 2.2   Older people, by sex, age group and family situation, Great Britain, 1991

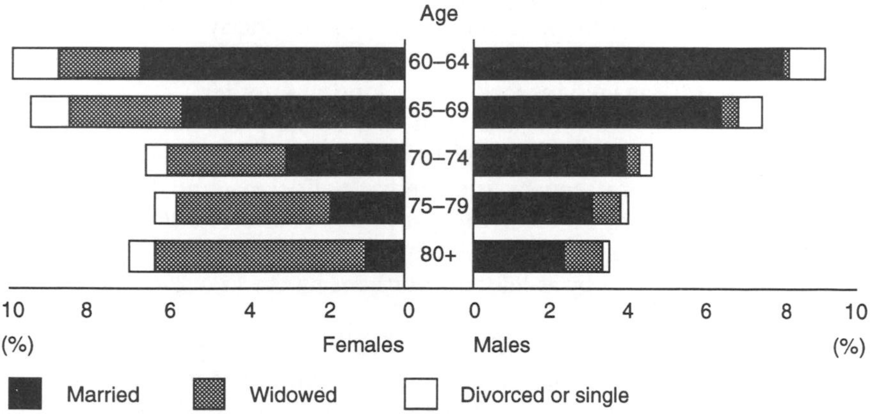

Source: Adapted from Family Policy Studies Centre/Centre for Policy on Ageing, Fact Sheet Special Edition, *Older People in the European Community* (1993), pp. 5–12.

But age is also of interest to sociologists as a social construction. The actual age of a person is given significance by the surrounding society and culture. For example, in most modern Western societies positions of power are held by people who are past the age of retirement. It is often said that even by the age of 50 most would find it difficult to gain employment and yet this is considered a young age for a person to become Prime Minister! Despite the upward trend in the mean age of women at childbirth (27.9 in 1994), woman in their early thirties although considered to be relatively young are frequently referred to as 'elderly primips' and treated with caution.

Old age has only become a 'social problem' in the latter half of this century for it was only then that it became a mass phenomenon. But older people as a group are just as fragmented by social class, ethnicity and gender as any other age group. It is older middle-class people in receipt of private pensions who are often the ones who are featured in advertisements for holidays and expensive retirement developments. The higher incidence of poverty is to be found among the group who throughout their lives have been the most vulnerable: working-class women. But even here, some may find that they have more money to spend on themselves in older age than was available throughout their lives. Among ethnic minorities as we have seen the numbers of elderly people are small but ethnicity too has a significance for their life-chances and experiences (Blakemore and Boneham, 1993).

Gender is obviously of great significance when studying the life-styles of older people as women's lives are not so affected by retirement from paid work as are men's. Women tend to continue to do household tasks, look after grandchildren and keep more contact with families than do men. Women are also more likely to be in some form of employment after the age of 60 than are men. This is particularly true of women who work in family-owned businesses, in agricultural communities, and as carers. This picture of gender differences in life-styles is rather accurately portrayed in the TV series 'Last of the Summer Wine', where elderly men are allowed to behave rather as schoolboys without responsibilities and the women of their age are still engaged in work of one kind or another.

As well as old age, youth is also seen as a 'social problem' – could it be that the group which has the power to define itself is middle-aged? Young 'teenage' mothers are seen by the media, politicians, and health-policy-makers as a 'problem', one of the proposals of the *Health of the Nation* (DOH, 1992) document was to reduce the numbers of conceptions amongst the under-16s by at least 50 per cent by the year 2000 (see Table 2.5).

Another problem associated with youth is unemployment. Youth unemployment is on as large a scale as unemployment in older age groups. Both age-sets tend to be defined as 'dependents' of the state and a social problem. This pattern of 'structured dependency' sociologists

Table 2.5 Live births, Great Britain, by age of mother, 1941–91

Age of mother (years) Year	15–19	20–24	25–29	30–34	35–39	40–44	45–49	All births (= 100%) (000)
1941	4.3	25.4	31.1	22.1	12.7	4.2	0.3	669
1951	4.3	27.6	32.2	20.7	11.5	3.4	0.2	768
1961	7.2	30.8	30.7	18.8	9.6	2.7	0.2	912
1971	10.6	36.5	31.4	14.1	5.8	1.5	0.1	870
1981	9.0	30.9	34.0	19.7	5.3	1.0	0.1	704
1991	7.6	24.8	35.6	23.0	7.6	1.2	0.1	766

Source: Adapted from OPCS, General Register Office (Scotland).

(Walker, 1980; Phillipson, 1982) argue is caused by exclusion from the production process and thus from economic rewards. Categorisation and definitions of age are then a social construct. For motherhood to be made possible for women of 60 has recently become a controversial subject as the result of IVF developments, but fatherhood for men of the same age is a cause for congratulation. It is the culture of society itself which determines the appropriateness of certain behaviour patterns and activities to a chronological age.

Sociologists seek to classify and identify certain social groups which share specific characteristics. This is applied in social research in order to further knowledge of the workings of society and in social policy to direct more accurately scarce resources to those in most need. The social divisions so far identified must be seen as a mesh of interconnecting threads which are woven throughout modern society. There are other factors too, such as mental and physical disability and also the geographical location in which many of these divisions become centred. We now look at two areas in which these divisions can be seen most clearly: poverty and health.

■ Poverty

Social researchers first began to measure the extent of poverty in the nineteenth century. The studies by Booth in the east end of London and Rowntree in York were the first to attempt to set a poverty line by which differing grades of poverty could be calculated. Other studies at this time illustrated the cost of food, rent and necessities for a family on low income (Pember Reeves, 1911). This interest by social researchers in the extent and causes of poverty affected social legislation and influenced the direction of social work in the twentieth century.

The measurement and definition of poverty has changed throughout this time, and is still changing. How can poverty be defined in modern industrial societies ? The division is made between *absolute* poverty which is usually defined as living below a basic subsistence level such as that which appertains in some areas of the developing world today and in some parts of Britain in the last century and this. But today, most sociologists and researchers talk of *relative* poverty as being a more useful concept. Peter Townsend has most clearly defined this idea of poverty being related to a person's surrounding community and social networks:

> Individuals, families and groups in the population can be said to be in poverty when they lack the resources to obtain the types of diet, participate in the activities and have the living conditions and amenities which are customary, or at least widely encouraged or approved, in the societies to which they belong. (Townsend, 1979, p. 31)

The problem with trying to define poverty objectively is, of course, that ideas of 'average' living standards are vague and people find it difficult to agree on what constitutes deprivation. In the 1980s, researchers working on a survey of *Breadline Britain* gained a two-thirds consensus from a public opinion survey that the following indices represented necessities for an acceptable standard of living:

* self-contained accommodation with indoor toilet and bath;
* weekly roast joint and three meals a day for children;
* money for public transport;
* heating and carpets;
* toys for children;
* money for Christmas;
* and a refrigerator and washing machine. (Mack and Lansley, 1985)

However, the definition of what constitutes poverty still remains a matter of debate; in the *Social Attitudes Survey* (Taylor-Gooby, 1990) only 25 per cent were prepared to agree with the Townsend definition of relative poverty, with 50 per cent agreeing with a more 'breadline' definition, but there was a near-unanimous agreement (92 per cent) on a definition of poverty as 'not having enough to eat without getting into debt' – a near-absolute or below subsistence definition.

Statistics on poverty are very complex to analyse as the definition of poverty which is used can differ and thus alter calculations. The definition used in government statistics before 1988 was that of 'low income families' (LIF), but this was abandoned in favour of the 'households below average income' (HBA) scale. By calculating households instead of families the number of persons constituting this group became of great significance. The statistical effect was to reduce the number of people living on 'below

Figure 2.3 Percentage of people whose income is below selected fractions of average income, before housing costs, 1961–92

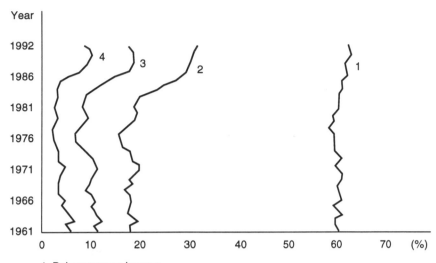

1 Below average income
2 Below 60% of everage income
3 Below half average income
4 Below 40% of average income

Sources: Adapted from *Social Trends*, 25 (1995).

half the average income' by over a million. But in calculating the numbers in the total population living on the unofficial 'poverty line' of below average income, we can see that the total rose during the 1980s (Figure 2.3).

By 1995 it was reported that a third of all households (27 per cent of all families), were in receipt of some form of means-tested benefits. In other words, they were deemed by official calculations to be entitled to benefits by virtue of the fact that their income was below the minimum level (Figure 2.4).

☐ **Social composition, location and causes of poverty**

The groups most likely to be poor are:

• families with dependent children;
• lone mothers;
• disabled people;
• single pensioners (especially females).

Children are the main cause of poverty for women alone and for couples. We will look at the policies and benefits payable to tackle family poverty in

Figure 2.4 The growth of dependency: number of recipients
of means-tested benefits, 1979–94

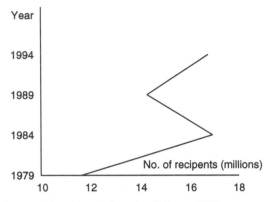

Sources: Adapted from *Independent* (8 August 1995).

Chapter 6. The poor are most likely to be in rented accommodation both public and private, to be unemployed, to have no access to a car or telephone and to be entirely dependent upon such benefits. This relatively high incidence of poverty in families with dependent children means that many ethnic minorities are over-represented among the poor. Over 66 per cent of Pakistani and Bangladeshi and over 50 per cent of Indian families are couples with dependent children, compared with only 20 per cent of white families. Among the Afro-Caribbean population the incidence of single mothers is relatively high and this coupled with the fact that most families will contain more than two dependent children makes them more 'at risk' from poverty (see Figure 2.5).

The higher incidence of poverty in certain areas therefore is likely to be connected to factors of social composition, public housing and unemployment. But it should not be forgotten that some areas of poverty may be surrounded by comparative affluence. An area such as Camden in London, for example, contains some of the most concentrated areas of poverty and wealth. Poverty is fragmented and dispersed but it can also be more concentrated than wealth. In the South Wales valleys there is a large extent of poverty but it may not be so concentrated as in other urban areas. The areas of Britain with the most widespread poverty are South Wales, Scotland and the north-east of England, whereas the south-east and East Anglia are areas of widespread wealth.

Within large areas there are pockets of poverty, many of them concentrated on so-called 'sink' estates which have become the housing offered to lone mothers, ethnic minorities and large families on benefits, as well as some disabled or mentally ill people. These estates frequently become stigmatised and only those who are powerless to command any alternative will accept a place there. Other areas of poverty concentration

Figure 2.5 People in poverty, below 40 per cent of average income, before housing costs, 1961–89

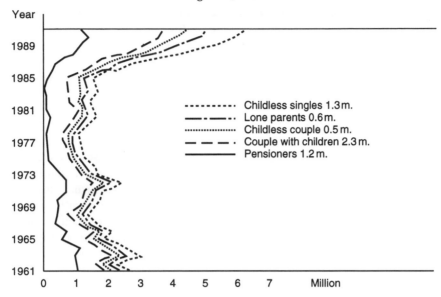

Sources: Adapted from *Independent* (3 June 1994).

can be found in the older properties in inner cities, especially those which have been deserted by industry, this is especially significant for ethnic minorities. People from ethnic minorities live almost exclusively in urban and former manufacturing areas of inner cities. Although home-ownership is relatively high among the Asian population, the houses owned tend to be terraced properties built before 1919 and lacking modern amenities. The poor therefore tend to be segregated (Smith, 1987), and this often means a racial as well as social segregation. The causes of poverty have also been debated since the studies of the nineteenth century. Basically the suggested causes are seen as either structural – that is, due to social and economic forces in society, or personal – that is, due to an inadequacy of the poor themselves. Most sociological studies have focused upon the structural causes: unemployment, low wages, racial disadvantage, ill-health. There have been studies which have attempted to define a culture of poverty (Lewis, 1964) which argues that the attitudes, beliefs and values of the poor themselves are both a cause and an effect of poverty.

This argument has been used to explain the persistence of poverty from one generation to another. This is the cycle-of-poverty debate which sees poverty as almost an inheritable characteristic of people rather than structures. Undoubtedly children who are born to families living in poverty are more likely to be in poverty in adult life and so a certain cyclical pattern is observable, but is this because of personal failings or the structures of society? This debate has resonances of 'nature' versus 'nurture' which we have examined in respect of gender and ethnicity. As we have discussed, the current debate concerning the construction of a marginalised underclass of the dependent poor (Murray, 1990) also focuses upon a specific set of values which are said to be instrumental in creating this group.

Poverty represents the extreme illustration of a socially divided society but studies of the nation's health also show the effect of social divisions.

☐ Health inequalities

The chances of people living a long and healthy life are also structured by factors of social class and poverty, ethnicity and, of course, gender. In many ways it is quite difficult to compare the relative health status of males and females as they are obviously vulnerable at different stages in their lives to different diseases, potential risk and biological factors which influence mortality and morbidity rates. The saying 'men die and women get sick' appears to be borne out by health statistics. Life expectancy for men is, on average, 74 years whilst for women it is 80 years. Men, especially under the age of 30, are twice as likely as women to die a violent death either by accident or suicide. But it must be remembered that these are general statistics and contain great differences between social classes and ethnic groups.

The main area of health where gender is said to be a factor is in the greater diagnosis of women as suffering from some form of mental illness. Many more women than men are admitted to psychiatric institutions, this of course illustrates the number who have been officially diagnosed as mentally ill. (For statistics of hospital admissions see Table 2.7.)

As can be seen, apart from greater male vulnerability to drug and alcohol dependency and schizophrenia, mental illness – especially forms of depression – is far more prevalent in women. The incidence of more older women in the population and of post-natal depression does of course increase the figures but does not explain such a great sex difference. A sociological explanation of this phenomenon focuses upon three main perspectives:

- social causation;
- social and cultural labelling;
- anomaly of the measuring methodology. (Pilgrim and Rogers, 1993)

In other words, many writers (Brown and Harris, 1978) argue that it is the role of women within the private domestic sphere which renders them more liable to suffer from depression. Others (Pilgrim and Rogers, 1993; Williams *et al.*, 1986) argue that women are more likely than men to consult a doctor because of emotional stress. Joan Busfield (1982) argued

Table 2.6 Rates of admission to hospitals per 100 000 population, by sex and diagnostic group, England, 1986

Diagnosis	Male	Female	Excess of female over over male rate
All diagnoses	364	468	+29
Schizophrenia	66	58	−12
Affective psychoses	35	68	+98
Other psychoses	32	44	+37
Senile and presenile dementia	33	55	+67
Alcohol psychoses and alcoholism	45	20	−55
Drug dependence	9	8	−11
Neurotic disorders	22	42	+91
Personality and behaviour disorders	28	32	+14
Other conditions*	89	142	+60
Rates for all diagnoses (1986)	364	468	+29
Rates for all diagnoses (1976)	320	447	+40

* Includes depression not classified elsewhere.
Source: Pilgrim and Rogers (1993), p. 23. Reproduced by permission.

that the figures are skewed because of the exclusion of some forms of mental illness such as personality disorders and some organic conditions which would show that more men than supposed suffer from mental illness. However research by Gove (1983) purported to show that marital status was an important variable with married women being more likely than married men or single women to suffer from mental illness. Busfield (1982) also argued that single men were hospitalised more often than married women. Other feminist writers (Ehrenreich and English, 1973; Chesler, 1972) put forward the view that women are more likely to be 'labelled' as mentally and emotionally unstable by the male psychiatric establishment. These sociological perspectives are also applied to explanations of the greater reported incidence of hospital admissions for mental illness among the 'black' ethnic groups. Although the data collection methods and definitions of mental illness must be treated with reservations nevertheless the overall picture is one of the over-representation of Afro-Caribbean and South Asian people in the hospitalisation statistics. Afro-Caribbeans males are five times more likely, and Asian males three times more likely, to be diagnosed as schizophrenic than are whites (Bhat *et al.*, 1988). Afro-Caribbeans are also more likely to be labelled as 'aggressive' and be subject to a sectioning order (Bhat *et al.*, 1988).

The over-representation of both women and 'black' ethnic minorities in the diagnosis and admissions for mental illness is well-researched and the subject of great sociological discussion and debate. The role of inequality, prejudice and discrimination as a possible causation or misdiagnosis is the most frequently-used sociologically-based explanation.

Women, of course, compose the greater number of hospital admissions and GP consultations, but this must be seen against the background of the almost 100 per cent hospitalisation of childbirth, the antenatal attendance at both GP and hospital clinics and the fact that it is women who are most likely to accompany babies and children to see a doctor. It is this responsibility for children's and family health and the expectation that it is women who will provide care for the sick at home, which is said to lead to higher rates of female absences from work and not the fact that women are more likely to be ill themselves. But, as with race and ethnicity the impact of social and economic class and poverty on differential rates of health and illness is probably paramount.

There are social divisions and inequalities of health in modern Britain – this has been borne out by the *Black Report* (1982) and subsequent other research studies (Whitehead, 1988; Rowntree, 1995). Vulnerability to earlier death is greater in the lower social classes at all ages (see Figure 2.6).

For both women and men, deaths from heart disease, most cancers, and strokes are higher among the lower social classes (Whitehead, 1988). Only breast and ovarian cancer in women, and melanoma in both sexes showed a reverse trend. It is suggested that the higher incidence of breast and ovarian cancer in women of higher social classes, is related to childbearing patterns (Blackburn, 1991).

Even by the time of birth itself, the impact of social and economic deprivation is felt with perinatal and infant mortality rates higher among the lower social classes (see also Chadwick, 1994) (see Figure 2.7).

Babies born to mothers who were themselves not born in the UK but in the New Commonwealth, are more likely to be of low birthweight and also have higher perinatal and neonatal death rates than those of UK-born mothers. It has been calculated (Macfarlane, Mugford, Johnson and Garcia, 1995) that 6.6 per cent babies of UK-born mothers were of low birth-weight compared with 9.7 per cent of those whose mothers were born in the 'New Commonwealth'. However recent research shows that there is a wide variation within 'black' ethnic groups (Andrews and Jewson, 1993), with Bangladeshis exhibiting the lowest health status.

The childhood disease which is most directly associated with poverty is rickets. This disorder was prevalent in poor working-class areas of Britain before the Second World War but was almost eradicated in the post-war period. In the 1980s, there were many reports of this 'lost' disease among children and pregnant women in the Asian communities of the inner cities (Donovan, 1986; McNaught, 1988). But interestingly, from a

Figure 2.6   Occupational class mortality in babies and adults, early 1980s

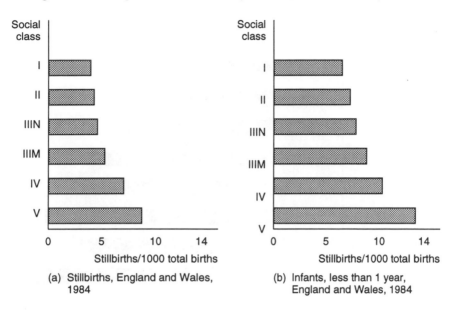

(a) Stillbirths, England and Wales, 1984

(b) Infants, less than 1 year, England and Wales, 1984

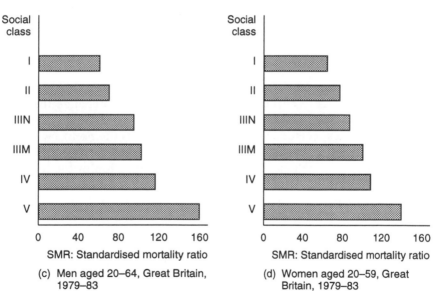

(c) Men aged 20–64, Great Britain, 1979–83

(d) Women aged 20–59, Great Britain, 1979–83

Sources: Adapted from OPCS (1986).

Figure 2.7   Low birth weight, by father's social class, England and Wales, 1992

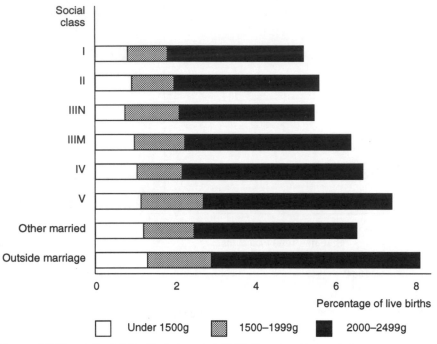

Sources: OPCS mortality statistics; Macfarlane *et al.* (1995). Reproduced by permission.

sociological perspective, the suggested remedy from many health educationalists was to encourage these communities to change their diet and life-style. Asian women were criticised for not following antenatal advice and the expectation was that it was the victims themselves who were at fault and had to change. This contrasts with the post-war measures taken to combat the disease among the white population by the fortifying of margarine with vitamins and the allocation of free school milk (Donovan, 1986). The 'victim-blaming' approach to health and behaviour is one which has become more prevalent in recent years. Some of the more extreme health education messages have often appeared to be blaming the individual for her/his own ill-health. This individualist perspective was most pronounced in *The Health of the Nation* (Department of Health, 1992) survey which failed to recognise the contribtory effects of poverty, unemployment and housing on rates of disease. The Winterton Report (House of Commons, 1992) on the future of maternity services did briefly mention the low income of some mothers and the consequent inadequacies of diet and housing which followed, but this was not taken up in the subsequent report of the Expert Maternity Group (DOH, 1993). 'Risky' behaviour such as smoking or eating an unhealthy diet are products of economic structures as well as individual or group 'choices'.

The Maternity Alliances' research has shown that many pregnant women on supplementary benefit are incapable of affording a healthy diet. The greater likelihood that women from ethnic minorities will live in deprived areas and be in poverty renders them more likely to suffer from an inadequate diet and low health standard. Equally, mothers in low income groups are more likely to smoke and less likely to breastfeed. The 1990 survey (OPCS) on breast-feeding showed that this continues to be a social-class-related activity. In Britain, older and more educated women were most likely to breast-feed, 78 per cent of babies from professional classes compared with only 51 per cent from manual workers' families. Behaviour such as smoking, eating unhealthy 'junk' food and refusing to breast-feed, although often classed by outsiders as irrational and ignorant may be interpreted quite differently by the people themselves. For those living in cramped, damp, overcrowded and deprived surroundings, these 'choices' represent ways in which they can better manage their lives.

The explanation for the differentials in health between social classes, ethnic groups and in some respects between males and females cannot be found in one simple overarching perspective. But people of low social classes, women and ethnic minorities are most likely to be in poverty and to suffer from low standards of health. This pattern is also likely to become generational. The explanation is probably to be found in a mixture of structural and cultural causes. A sociological perspective would of course view cultural beliefs and behaviour patterns as being themselves produced by economic and social factors.

☐ **Midwifery and poverty**

Many studies in midwifery and the social sciences consider the impact of social class, poverty and unemployment on pregnancy outcomes. MIDIRS (Midwives' Information and Resource Service) has a standard search entitled, 'Poverty/socioeconomic factors affecting pregnancy'. It is beyond the scope of this text to review all the relevant literature but the evidence of the adverse effects of poverty and deprivation on pregnancy outcomes is well-established.

According to the Department of Social Security (DSS, 1994) a quarter of the British population is now living on less than half the national average income. In 1988 the number of pregnant women on means tested benefits was one in five, by 1994 it had risen to one in three (the Maternity Alliance, 1995). Perinatal and infant mortality rates show a vast variation between countries and between regions. In the United Kingdom, in 1994 the stillbirth rate, for social class I was 4.2 which was almost half of that of social class V. The perinatal mortality rates for social class I was 6.3, whilst the rate for social class V was 8.9 (OPCS, 1994). 66 per cent of babies born to mothers on benefits had a birth weight below the national average and were at greater risk of ill health (OPCS, 1994, 1995). Whilst the information collected is incomplete, based on estimates and outdated definitions of social class, there are still many studies that record the impact and adverse effects of poverty and social deprivation on health. There is also growing research evidence on the correlation between morbidity in childbearing women and their offspring and poor maternal nutrition (Crawford, 1993; Pharoah et al., 1990). Mortality rather than morbidity is easily measured, and as a consequence the higher trends in morbidity associated with low socioeconomic status can be, and are easily ignored (Black et al., 1988; Whitehead, 1988; Law et al., 1993; Martyn, 1994; Wilkinson, 1994; Barker, 1995). The DSS (1994) provide evidence to support the fact that families with children, both couples and lone parents, are over represented at the bottom end of the income distribution with 57 per cent having a household income below 40 per cent of the UK average.

One of the most relevant studies is by Oakley et al. (1990). This study is important for many reasons. It considers the effects of poverty and also attempts to measure in a systematic way, the benefits of midwifery care. In this research 509 women who had already had a low birthweight baby were randomised either to receive standard antenatal care or care from a research midwife. The study population was socially disadvantaged:

77 per cent of the women were working class;
18 per cent had unemployed partners;
41 per cent smoked at booking.

The research midwives offered additional 'social support'. This included participating in a wide range of very different activities including listening to women and discussing their problems, obtaining advice about benefits, filling in forms, writing letters to housing departments, providing baby clothes, going with women to local support groups, taking animals to the vet and pursuing detailed medical questions raised by women (Oakley, 1994). The trial was conducted in four centres in England. Pregnancy outcomes were measured using information in the case notes and postal questionnaires. The results were extensive, far-reaching and of great interest to midwives. Babies in the social support group were heavier and there were fewer low birthweight babies. The women in this group were less likely to have their labour induced or to have epidurals. There were more spontaneous births. The infants that required resuscitation were similar in both groups but those in the supported group needed less invasive methods and less neonatal care. The babies were healthier in the early weeks and needed less medical care.

The authors conclude that social support can never compensate for the cumulative effects of social disadvantage but there were clear benefits when midwives 'listened to women'. Writing some three and a half years before the publication of Changing Childbirth (DOH, 1993), they conclude:

> Although the policy implications of our findings must be in the direction of promoting continuity of care and a less impersonal and more sensitive antenatal service, it is important to remember that social policy changes are also needed to improve the health-denying conditions in which many mothers and babies live. (Oakley *et al.*, 1990, pp. 155–61)

Another important study is the 'Newcastle Community Midwifery Care Project' (Davies and Evans, 1991) which was set up to provide enhanced support by midwives to childbearing women in their own home, in an area of the city defined as having a concentration of high-risk factors, and to measure the effects of this intervention. The interventions included more personal, individual contact, better advice on smoking, diet, access to services and benefits, parentcraft classes. The results were extensive and conclusive. Women were more likely to be satisfied with their care seeing it as more appropriate to their needs and they valued the close relationship they established with the midwife. The study also demonstrated that 'defaulting' (missing two or three clinic appointments) was not as great a problem as the anecdotal evidence suggested. The intervention of the midwives in the project had no effect on perinatal mortality nor on the incidence of abnormalities in the baby but there was important evidence of a reduced incidence of low birthweight babies. The numbers were small so the results should be treated with caution. There was a small reduction in the numbers of pre-term deliveries. The women in the project group used less pain relief in labour.

The benefits of reducing low birthweight are significant. The cost of treating such infants is usually measured in terms of financial cost – the psychological, emotional and physical costs to the family are difficult to count so tend not to be counted. The authors of this study conclude that despite the strength of the research evidence and the widespread agreement with the findings, there was considerable difficulty in securing funding to continue to offer this clearly beneficial style of midwifery care.

This chapter is probably one of the most important in this book. The major medical causes of mortality and morbidity have largely been eliminated, but poverty and deprivation still continue to claim the lives of disadvantaged women and their vulnerable babies.

Case Study 2.1

Helen is a community midwife working in a large urban area with a pleasant rural area to the north of the district. She does not work with any particular GP and most of her work is via the hospital antenatal clinic. She has been asked to visit two women in her area in order to conduct an 'antenatal assessment' and to arrange for community antenatal care. Helen is very experienced and sometimes conducts home births. She prefers the 'Domino scheme' (Domicilary in and out) and often escorts women into hospital for delivery. The GPs in the area are reluctant to be involved with intra partum care but are happy to run antenatal clinics in their surgeries.

Helen has two addresses in her diary today. The first she recognises as Marian whom she has met in her previous pregnancies.

Marian is single but lives most of the time with Charlie. Charlie sometimes disappears for weeks on end. Marian is now 20 years old and Charlie is probably about 30. Marian is not intelligent but manages to care for herself. She lives in a one-bedroomed Local Authority high-rise flat on the fifteenth floor. There is a lift but often it does not work. The flat is damp and is heated by electricity. There is an additional electric fire in the flat but two of the three elements are faulty. The electricity bills are very high and Marian uses the fire as little as possible. Marian is unemployed and lives on benefits. A proportion of her weekly income is deducted each week to pay for arrears on her fuel bills and in repayment of loans from the Social Fund. She is also hooked on the National Lottery and spends at least £2 per week on tickets. Her rent is paid directly to the local authority by Housing Benefit. Her diet is very poor. She eats mainly bread, biscuits and crisps. She rarely eats fresh fruit or vegetables and never buys fish, chicken or fresh meat. She does not drink alcohol at all. She is overweight and smokes around 10–15 cigarettes per day. She also has a large dog. Her boyfriend, Charlie, sometimes calls in with 'take away' meals and cigarettes especially when he has some money. This seems to follow periods away from home. The estate where Marian lives has a bus route into the town and has some small local shops. There is a free bus to a local supermarket which runs three times per week.

Marian is well-known to the community midwives. Her first two children were born after difficult pregnancies and were both of low birthweight. The first child, a son, was admitted to hospital on numerous occasions, failing to thrive and is now being cared for by foster parents. Her second child, also a boy, is also in local authority care with foster-parents. Marian sees her sons at least every month and now wants a daughter.

When Helen first meets Marian in this pregnancy she is just beginning to feel fetal movements and says she is well. She remembers Helen and invites her to stay for tea.

She looks pale, is tired and inadequately dressed. The flat is cold and damp.

Case Study 2.2

The next woman on Helen's case load is Vicky. Helen has already spoken to Vicky by telephone on three occasions after Vicky rang the antenatal clinic seeking advice. Helen had promised to visit as soon as possible that morning but had been delayed at Marian's flat. Vicky, a primary-school teacher, is married to Peter, a computer manager. They live in a large detached house in a rural area. They have a large garden, employ domestic help and have no pets. Vicky is 32 years old and pregnant for the first time. She and Peter have had a long history of treatment for infertility and had three unsuccessful attempts at In vitro fertilisation. They had the treatment at a private clinic. After the last unsuccessful attempt they decided to abandon treatment and resolve to live as a childless couple. Within two months Vicky was pregnant. It is the start of the long school summer holidays and Vicky is now twelve weeks pregnant. She has had a scan at the private hospital and all is well. She has been referred to the local maternity hospital and is anxious to meet Helen as soon as possible. She is extremely anxious. Her main concerns are that the baby will be adversely affected by the earlier fertility treatment, fear of labour and 'losing control', fear of spontaneous miscarriage and fear about most of the things her mother-in-law tells her are a risk. These include many of the old wives' tales such as eating strawberries leading to birth marks and stretching to peg out washing leading to strangling the baby with the umbilical cord. She has read widely on the subject of birth and has already written an extensive Birth Plan. She does not want any pharmacological pain relief in labour, she does not want Syntometrine, she does not want continuous fetal monitoring. The list is extensive and clear. It is obvious to Helen that Vicky has many unrealistic expectations and needs time to talk and to establish a good relationship with her midwife. Her main questions today are about the frequency and definition of fetal movements and about the research evidence on Sudden Unexplained Infant Death Syndrome. Vicky is physically very well, she has a good diet, sleeps well and enjoys regular exercise. The pregnancy is developing normally. She would like a Domino delivery because she has read that it is an effective method of achieving continuity of carer in her area where maternity care is still organised in a traditional way.

■ Questions and discussion points

- Whose needs are greater, Marian's or Vicky's? Justify your answer.
- Within the constraints of the system how can Helen, the midwife, best prioritise her care?
- How does disability (physical or mental) increase poverty?
- Has the Welfare State eliminated poverty? If not, why not?
- Debate Universalism (e.g. Child Benefit) and Selectivism (payments from the Social Fund) in providing welfare benefits. Should benefits be targeted to those in 'real need'? (See also Chapter 6)
- As these case studies show, social divisions and inequalities exist in all societies. How have sociologists analysed these divisions? How can understanding the explanations of inequality assist the midwife in giving better care?
- Why is Marian poor?
- Is poverty the fault of the poor?
- Are there ethical dilemmas in Helen's case-load? If so what are they and how can these be resolved?

Key points

- Sociologists attempt to explain divisions in society.
- The main factors of stratification are social class, race, ethnicity, gender and age.
- The Registrar-General Classification of Social Class is now considered to be an inappropriate model. Other scales are more useful in identifying specific clusters of deprivation.
- Studies of class culture are considered to be more useful in making sense of society.
- Ethnicity (rather than race) is used by sociologists as a measuring tool and as an explanation for patterns of inequality.
- Gender, not sex, is a social construct. Sociologists are interested in the persistence of inequalities in life chances for women.
- Sociology studies have demonstrated that age is one of the most important group characteristics in explanations of inequality.
- It is the culture of society that determines the appropriateness or otherwise of certain behaviour, e.g. it would appear that pregnancy is 'sensible' between the ages of 20 and 30, in marriage, where the husband is of a similar age to his wife and financially able to support his wife and child. There are few exceptions to these rules.
- Sociologists have defined absolute and relative poverty. In 1995, 33 per cent of all families were in receipt of some form of means-tested benefits.
- The groups most likely to be poor are: families with dependent children, lone mothers, disabled people and single female pensioners.
- The suggested causes of poverty are seen as structural (unemployment, low wages, poor housing, ill-health), or personal, when poverty is thought to be part of a cycle of deprivation and the fault of the poor.
- The chances of people living a long and healthy life are influenced by social class, poverty, ethnicity and gender.
- Many government health education messages appear to ignore the structural causes of poverty and instead blame the individual for his or her own ill-health.
- Breast-feeding continues to be an example of a social-class-related activity.

Chapter 3

Sociological perspectives on 'the family' and community

Midwives are concerned with families. They offer care to women in all types of families or family groups. If their care is to be thoughtful and helpful to women they need to understand more about the environment where care takes place. This chapter will be concerned with the unravelling of a dominant area of study in sociology which is also a part of everyday life and a basic organisation in most societies – the family. The idea of 'the family' is such a familiar one that it is nearly always used as a means of introducing students to the basic approach of sociology. It illustrates the way in which sociological theories and analyses can enrich but also problematise, and question accepted and seemingly simplistic aspects of everyday social life.

One thing becomes apparent when we review the sociology of 'the family' and that is that there is no such thing! The most important phrase which could be used to summarise sociological studies of families is that of *diversity*. A model of what is often termed 'the traditional family' consisting of the 'Janet and John' ideal – father the breadwinner, mother at home with dependent children, has been socially constructed in the British culture as the 'norm' which is either the truth or is a pattern to be aspired to. In reality, the overwhelming majority of the population in the final decade of the twentieth century live in many differing family types and formations.

■ When was 'the family'?

Very often rhetoric on 'the family' and 'community' tends to set up a vision of a lost golden age when everybody lived in stable families, no divorce, no domestic violence, no child abuse, no illegitimacy and women and men knew their place and did not question their roles. This, in fact, is an unlikely but untestable assumption. Changes in divorce legislation, in criminal proceedings, in the increased willingness of people to articulate problems and experiences has meant that it is impossible truly to compare 'the family' over time.

The fact that divorce rates, for instance, have increased over the past decades does NOT necessarily mean that people had happier marriages before 1970 when divorce was made easier to obtain for the majority of the population.

Social historians also differ in their views on the historical development of the family from an extended family to the 'modern' nuclear structure. Peter Laslett (1972), for instance has strenuously argued that the nuclear family was extremely common in pre-industrial Britain and was not a product of industrialisation. Others, like Shorter (1977) and ·Zaretsky (1976), have argued that the structure of family groups is constructed by the surrounding economic and social development. The development of industrial capitalism meant that the workforce needed to be more mobile and that the nuclear family was more suited to this type of economy than the extended networks which were more functional to a peasant and agricultural society which was more static.

Sociologists, especially in Britain during the period of the 1950s and 1960s, also concentrated on empirical studies of family structures in various regions and on social change in these structures (Wilmott and Young, 1960; Rosser and Harris, 1965; Fletcher, 1962). Much of this type of sociological study emphasised the regional and social class differences in family structures. In their study of Bethnal Green in the 1950s, Wilmott and Young argued that it was at this historical juncture that the working-class pattern of extended family networks was being replaced by fragmentation into nuclear families among a younger generation. Many studies of Britain in this period (Goldthorpe and Lockwood, 1968; Bott, 1957) continued this theme of changing social patterns. The over-whelming view was that the pattern of the nuclear family which was characteristic of the rising middle classes in the latter part of the nineteenth century was now being adopted by the working class in the affluent post-war period (Sennett, 1977). As we shall see in Chapter 7, social policies after 1945 did assume that the nuclear family was the norm upon which subsequent policies were based.

Sociology at this time, tended to describe changes in family structures but to accept that 'the family' existed as a social institution and it was as a system that it was studied. As we shall see in Chapter 5, more critical and feminist studies of family life and of the roles played by women and men within it appeared in the 1980s (Barrett and McIntosh, 1982).

In order to understand the changing view taken by sociologists on the role of 'the family' it is important to see how family structures have changed between the 1960s and the 1990s, the most significant change being the increase in single mothers.

■ Families today

As can be seen in Table 3.1 the number of people living alone has greatly increased and so have the number of lone parents, whilst the 'traditional'

Table 3.1 People in households, by type of household and family in which they live, Great Britain, 1961–92, per cent

Household type / Year	Living alone	Married couple, NC	Married couple, DC*	Married couple, NDC	Lone parent, DC*	Other house-holds	All people in private households** (= 100%) (000)
1961	3.9	17.8	52.2	11.6	2.5	12.0	49 545
1971	6.3	19.3	51.7	10.0	3.5	9.2	52 347
1981	8.0	19.5	47.4	10.3	5.8	9.0	52 760
1991	10.7	23.0	41.1	10.8	10.0	4.3	54 056
1992	11.1	23.4	39.9	10.9	10.1	4.6	

NC   No children.

DC   With dependent children.

NDC   With non-dependent children only.

*   These family types may also include non-dependent children.

**   1961, 1971, 1981 and 1991 Census data; 1992 General Household Survey.

Source: Adapted from General Register Office (Scotland); *Social Trends, 24* (1994), p. 34.

family has declined. The increase in divorce, and also in the number of single (i.e. never married) women who choose to be mothers but not wives, largely accounts for the increase in lone parents, whilst the increased numbers of elderly people (mostly female) contributed to the increase in single households.

As can be seen in Table 3.2, divorce rates have risen steadily since 1971 (see Chapter 6) and Britain now has the highest divorce rate in the EC, matched only by Denmark. The highest rates of divorce now occur among younger people aged under 30 who have been married for less than 10 years. Divorced or separated women are more likely to cohabit than to remarry, so although marriage may be less popular and divorce rates increasing, there still appears to be a trend towards setting up a family group.

Most divorce rates show the end of first marriages, although it should be noted that the number of failed remarriages has risen to 17 per cent for women and 18 per cent for men in 1991 (Family Policy Bulletin, 1991). One result of younger people divorcing is that according to the latest OPCS estimate, one in four children under the age of 16 will experience their parents' divorce (see Table 3.2).

Has the number of births outside marriage increased over the past century? The only truthful answer is that we do not know! We can compare rates for the past fifty years with a reasonable degree of accuracy

Table 3.2 Divorce, by sex and age, England and Wales,
per 1000 married population, 1961–91

	1961	*1971*	*1981*	*1991*
Females				
16–24	2.4	7.5	22.3	27.7
25–29	4.5	13.0	26.7	31.3
30–34	3.8	10.5	20.2	25.1
35–44	2.7	6.7	14.9	17.2
45 and over	0.9	2.8	3.9	4.5
All aged 16 and over	2.1	5.9	11.9	13.4
Males				
16–24	1.4	5.0	17.7	25.9
25–29	3.9	12.5	27.6	32.9
30–34	4.1	11.8	22.8	28.5
35–44	3.1	7.9	17.0	20.1
45 and over	1.1	3.1	4.8	5.6
All aged 16 and over	2.1	5.9	11.9	13.6

Source: Adapted from *Social Trends*, 24 (1994).

Table 3.3 Conceptions, by marital status and outcome, England and Wales, 1971–91, per cent

	1971	1981	1990	1991
Outside marriage				
Maternities inside marriage	8.1	5.5	3.9	3.7
Maternities outside marriage*				
joint registration	3.5	6.8	17.6	18.9
sole registration	4.1	4.8	6.2	6.1
Legal abortions**	6.7	11.4	15.5	15.0
Inside marriage				
Maternities	72.6	65.9	52.3	51.9
Legal abortions**	5.2	5.6	4.4	4.4
All conceptions				
(= 100%) (000)	835.5	752.3	871.5	853.7

* Births outside marriage can be registered by the mother only (sole registrations) or by both parents (joint registrations).

** Legal terminations under 1967 Abortion Act.

Source: Adapted from *Social Trends*, 24 (1994).

but we cannot project back into the past to compare like with like. The rates of illegitimacy in the Victorian age was largely a hidden figure, so too were reports of child abuse and infanticide, of domestic violence and of adultery. So we must be rigorous in our use of statistics on changing family structures and 'values'. For instance, despite the media publicity surrounding teenage mothers in the 1990s, the total number of teenage births was actually higher in the 1960s, with the numbers falling throughout the 1970s and 1980s (from 86 746 in 1966 to 47 900 in 1992). The numbers of pre-marital conceptions among teenage women has also fallen dramatically, from 35 793 in 1967 to 3 267 in 1992 (Selman, 1994). What has changed however is the response of society and women themselves to the incidence of teenage conception. In the 1960s and 1970s it was the norm for a premarital conception to be 'solved' by marriage – the so-called 'shot-gun wedding'. In 1971, 42 per cent of all births to married teenagers resulted from a premarital conception, but by 1991, 65 per cent of all extramarital births to teenage mothers were however, jointly registered. This points to the decline in forced marriages but an increase in cohabitation and joint registration of births. The main change for single mothers has been the rejection of marriage but the greater incidence of cohabitation, and also the greater likelihood of the mother 'keeping' the child rather than opting for adoption. Childbearing and cohabitation outside marriage have increased greatly in the past 15 or so years, in 1979 only 3 per cent of single women were cohabiting but by 1990 nearly 30 per cent were doing so. Births outside marriage currently represent about 33 per cent of all births.

The increase in lone parenting, the falling birth rate and the rise in legal terminations, has meant that the availability of babies for adoption has been drastically reduced.

Step-families are an increasing development of younger divorces, and have been the subject of a research study which reached some controversial conclusions (Kiernan, 1992). The results of this study conducted on children born in 1958, suggested that children living in step-families are more likely to leave home early, for girls to become pregnant before the age of 20, and for boys to leave school without qualifications. The tendency was, the study suggests, for children of step-families to be more 'at risk' than those from lone-parent families. Kathleen Kiernan's research points to the continuing increase in step-families, with divorces occurring at younger ages and it is estimated that 2.5 million children are today (1995) growing up in step-families.

The incidence of all types of lone-parent families also has a social class and ethnic significance which has ramifications for analyses of families in poverty (see Figure 3.1 and Chapter 2).

Figure 3.1 Lone-parent families, Great Britain, 1991

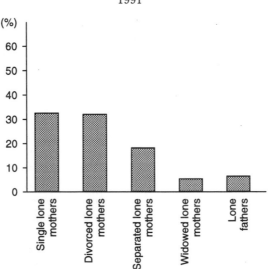

Sources: Adapted from *Guardian*, Educational Supplement (11 January 1994); *Haskey Population Trends* (1993).

■ 'Ethnic minority' families

One of the greatest social changes in Britain since 1945 has been the construction of Britain from a Colonial white society to a multicultural one, this has meant that *ethnicity* as well as social class must be a variable in any analysis of family structures (see Figure 3.2).

The interesting picture which emerges from these figures is that many black and Asian people are less likely than the white population to be in single-person households but that Asian families conform more closely to the 'ideal' of the close-knit family groups than do those of the indigenous white population.   On the other hand, West Indian women form the highest percentage of lone mothers. Among the 'white' population the highest number of single households (approximately 30 per cent of the total) are made up of people of pensionable age. Among the 'black' population however a higher number of single households (33 per cent) are made up of younger people, mainly single mothers. The rates of lone motherhood have been higher among the West Indian/Caribbean population for the past twenty years and this position remains.

What is the relationship between family size and other social factors? Historically, the birth rate in Britain has always shown an inverse social class ratio,.i.e. the higher the social class the lower the birth rate. It was the professional middle classes who first began limiting their families and this pattern remains although it is far less significant.

The greater participation of Afro-Caribbean women in the full-time workforce is often seen as an illustration of the more matriarchal power

Figure 3.2   Average household size, by ethnic group of head of household, Great Britain, 1991

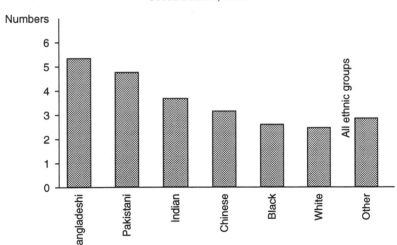

Sources: Adapted from *Social Trends*, 24 (1994); *General Household Survey*.

Figure 3.3 Lone mothers as percentage of all mothers, by ethnic group. Great Britain, 1989–91

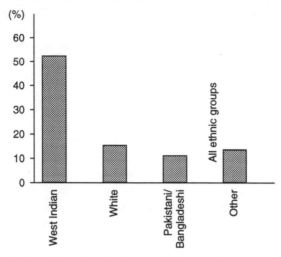

Sources: Adapted from Employment Department; *Social Trends*, 24 (1994)

structure of the Afro-Caribbean family. Writers such as Barrow (1982) have stressed the complex nature of different family forms in the Caribbean with both the 'common law' household based upon a long-term but unmarried relationship and the 'mother household' in which a woman (often the maternal grandmother) is the nominal family head. This pattern of female-headed families, it has been suggested, was also adopted by Afro-Caribbean women in Britain who looked to other women for child-care support (Wallerstein and Kelly, 1980).

The picture which emerges from this plethora of statistical information is of a society which is rich in diversity of family structures. There is not one model of 'the family' but many different formations within which people live a 'family life'.

Sociology then pinpoints this diversity of family structures over time and within British society at the present, the diverse nature of processes within family life and the significance of these for the lives of men and women. Of course, there is not one, but many sociological theories and emphases on the function and social meaning given to 'the family' in society.

Sociological theories of the family fall into two main categories; those which are concerned with the function of the family to the existence of society as a whole (Functionalist and Marxist), and those predominantly feminist accounts, which look at the internal workings of the family and in particular at the gender roles and inequalities which are produced within the site of the family. Others have been more concerned with looking at the family as an ideological formation which is used culturally to reproduce sets of social, gender and class relations of inequality (Gittins, 1985).

■ The family as a social structure

The externally orientated theories have defined the family as a *unit* and placed it in relation to the reproduction of both the values of society and the economic system. Both Marxist and functionalist accounts have tended to view the family as a unit of production in this way.

Talcot Parsons saw the family as having the function of the socialisation of children into the values and norms of society. It was the family which, he argued, was the primary socialisation agency and therefore was essential to the stability of society as a whole. His image of the family was one based very much on the strictly segregated roles of men and women. Women as mothers had the 'affective' role of providing emotional support, taking responsibility for the caring of children and elderly members and being a moral guide and educator. Men as fathers had the 'instrumental' role of the financial provider and were the predominant authority figures. This functionalist view put the stability of the family and its function to society as most important and was not really concerned with the effect of such prescriptive and proscriptive roles on the lives of individual men and women. This sociological view is one which came to be the projected 'norm' for family formation in both the USA and Britain and was the focus of much feminist criticism by the 1960s.

The classical Marxist view of the family was as a unit of production for the capitalist enterprise. It was within the family that the essentially capitalist values of personal possession and ownership was learned. The most famous Marxist text on the role of the family was that of Engels (1978), who theorised about the power relations within both bourgeois and proletarian family structures. He argued that the family with its structural exploitation of women was the basis of private property and capitalism. Bourgeois women were in a position of slavery without any control over their lives, they did not even own their own bodies but were simply for the reproduction and inheritance of bourgeois wealth and power. Proletarian women, on the other hand, existed in two spheres, they were slaves at home but were part of the industrial proletariat in the workplace. He saw the fact that the male worker could be compensated for his exploitation by the bourgeoisie at work by exploiting his wife at home, as a great barrier to the adoption of a radical class-consciousness. In many ways, Engels was the first to theorise that the family was consigned into the 'private' sphere of social life, and was instrumental in female inequality. The separation of industrial production from the domestic sphere and the placing of women in the domestic and out of

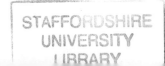

mainstream production process he called 'the classic defeat of the female sex'.

The American writer Veblen (1975) took up the Weberian theme of the importance of the bourgeois family as a unit of *consumption* in late nineteenth century capitalism. In a study of the 'conspicuous' flaunting of wealth and privilege among the newly wealthy in America, he defined the role of women in these families as the means by which wealth could be advertised. The role of women within the family was to wear the jewels and expensive clothes and be the hostess in mansions which would be a testament to the success of their husbands. This, argued Veblen, meant that women had only a vicarious status which was earned through their association with men: women not only advertised the status of men, they were 'status symbols' themselves. This definition of women as mere appendages to male status remained within the official categorisation of socio-economic class in social surveys, where women are assigned the position accruing to their husband or father.

The view of the family as being an economic unit of *production* was taken up in recent years by Marxist–feminist writers such as Christine Delphy (1984). She criticised the classical Marxist analyses as laying too much emphasis on roles in industrial production and ignoring the role of women in the *reproduction* of labour power. She saw the domestic role of women as an integral part of the capitalist system of production not as a private sphere outside the economic process. The domestic role was to reproduce labour power by the socialisation of future generations of workers, and women were an unpaid labour force which serviced the needs of workers. This placed domestic labour within the home firmly within the economic system and also recognised the gender division of labour power within the family.

■ The family as a social process

Although functionalists such as Parsons had long recognised that the family had an essential role as a social process, it was feminist sociologists, social psychologists and commentators who connected the socialisation role of the family specifically to the issue of female subordination. A feminist perspective shone the spotlight on the 'private' arena of the family and revealed that far from being the haven for women that it was often depicted, it was the site of exploitation and repression. As Lynne Segal (1983) has shown, however, feminism as a body of thought has been divided on the role of the family and its implications for women. For while some of the early writers saw the family as totally repressive and exploitative of women, some later writers saw it as a celebration of female power and authority which has not been recognised by society.

It seems axiomatic today to say that studies of the family automatically involve studies of gender roles, but this appeared as quite a revolutionary idea within sociology even at the beginning of the 1970s. Ann Oakley's proposal to research into the sociology of housework was rejected totally at first as it was not deemed to be a matter of any significance.

The idea that gender was a cultural definition as distinct from sex, which was a biological identity, had been illustrated by the anthropological studies of Margaret Mead (1943) and was taken up by sociology in the 1970s. This emphasis on gender as learned behaviour and not as a 'natural' and biological ascription excited the attention of feminist sociologists as it held out the potential for change and liberation for women. The great debate on 'nature *v.* nurture' dominated sociological studies of gender throughout the 1970s. Anne Oakley (1985) chronicled the different ways in which boys and girls are treated from babyhood and presented descriptions of cases where boy and girl androgynous twins, received differential gender upbringing which resulted in the adoption of male and female identities. (Androgynous, i.e. having the characteristics of both male and female: in these cases a decision has to be made to bring up the child as either a girl or boy.)

Studies of ways in which girls and boys were depicted in children's books and by toy-makers showed that girls were encouraged to be passive and boys were encouraged to be active. The positive attitudes of parents and especially of mothers to their male as opposed to relatively negative attitudes towards their female children became a subject of intense interest. It was in the family as the primary agent of socialisation that gender roles were learned and internalised. The internal power structures and practices of the family interested feminists as this posed an alternative view to the family as an homogeneous unit.

Those feminists who were critical of the family as a societal structure emphasised the inequality of power within the family setting. The early socialisation into gender roles resulted in the unequal distribution of economic resources and the segregation of male and female responsibilities. This segregation of conjugal roles meant that women took on the bulk of the burden of family life.

Women, it was argued (Finch and Groves, 1983) were socialised into becoming 'natural' carers and so the main responsibility for not only child-care but also care of spouses and relatives was disproportionately placed upon them. Women were therefore designated to the caring role which was economically unrewarded and also potentially mentally and physically destructive. Studies of mental illness showed that rates were highest for married women and single men and lowest for single women and married men (Brown and Harris, 1978). The prime responsibility for child-care and 'mothering' was also designated to women within the family and this too was criticised for restricting women's economic power rendering them dependent upon the male breadwinner.

But there was a strand of feminist work which argued that mothering was the basis of a female power base within the family which should be celebrated and emphasised. Writers such as Phyllis Chesler (1990) argue that there is a 'sacred bond' which biologically ties mother and child, and others (Kitzinger, 1978) posit what could be termed an 'earth-mother' image arguing for the essentialist nature of women and of the potential for women as mothers to find their true sphere of power within the family. Even Marxist–feminist writers such as Jane Humphries (1977) have put a more positive view of the family, viewing it as a working-class defence organisation against capitalist exploitation, but what a feminist perspective has enabled sociology to do is to analyse the basis of power and authority within the family.

■ Power structures within the family

As we saw in Chapter 1, there are contrasting sociological theoretical explanations for the bases of power and authority within society. When looking at the ways in which the family 'unit' was divided by power structures, there have been two principle explanations, economic and/or cultural.

But who has power and authority within the family? Is the family the one area of unchallenged female power, the site of matriarchal authority? Or does the family represent an area of patriarchal authority based upon greater access to economic resources by men? Before looking at these debates there is one point which is essential to bear in mind, the family structure which is assumed in many arguments is that of the white nuclear family. But as will become clear, even within this narrow definition, differences of social and economic class become apparent.

Before attempting to answer the question 'who has power within the family?' we must recognise that power relations are very complex. The division of labour within the family will to some extent determine the areas of authority of men and women. Some men have a degree of dependence upon women for cooking, washing and ironing and will admit to being 'useless' without them. Male helplessness and relative powerlessness in the domestic sphere is chronicled by writers such as Chris Lewis (1986). Some men may therefore experience a contradiction between being the 'master' but at the same time, pushed to the periphery in the family.

As Charles and Kerr (1988) have shown, it is women who make the everyday decisions on what food a family will consume and they also have the sole responsibility for the buying and cooking, but is this real authority or just management?

The woman's role as manager of the household resources especially in lower income groups has often been focused upon as an example of the home-based power of mothers. But recent studies (Wilson, 1989; Brannen and Moss, 1987) have shown that although they manage the scarce resources it is the men who decide on the distribution of the household income. When money becomes in scarce supply it is often the portion distributed by them to women and channelled then to children, which is cut. The fact that many women become objectively better-off financially as single parents (Graham, 1987) is a testament to their previous lack of control over resources.

Jan Pahl (1989) in her study of the distribution of income within families, constructed a typology of distribution and management which illustrated the significance of women's economic dependence. The management role (male as sole earner) was more prominent in lower income groups, the joint account (male main earner) was more indicative of lower middle class or affluent working-class groups, the joint account (shared accounts with both contributing) was of middle-class groups, the separate independent (both high earners but with segregated areas of responsibility) was true of older professional couples and homosexual pairings. Pahl argued therefore, that the amount of income and its distribution was inextricably linked to positions of power within the home but had its foundation in earning capacity outside the home.

For Marxist and functionalist explanations, the patriarchal nature of the family was based upon the dominating economic power of the male breadwinner. It was female economic dependence on men which was the basis for the family power structures. This is also the argument of many feminist writers who see women's disadvantaged economic position as the key to their subordination.

'Family' women have been entering the paid labour force in greater and greater numbers over the past twenty years, but they tend to be concentrated in the low-status, part-time and low-paid jobs (see Figure 3.4).

Even when women have paid employment outside the home however, there is evidence that men's share in domestic labour does not increase an appreciable amount but it is women's leisure time which is curtailed (see Table 3.4).

As Witherspoon and Prior (1991) noted: 'whatever talk there is of the "New Man", he is much rarer than the "New Woman"'. Even the higher visibility of men in day-to-day child care can be deceptive as analyses of the content of that care illustrate. Studies have shown that men tend to be able to choose which tasks to do, and take on those which are more pleasant and less time-consuming, for example, playing with children but not toileting them (La Rossa and La Rossa, 1981). This of course, places the whole debate on the basis of power back to the beginning, for if men have the power to choose which tasks to do, which food to eat, how money is to be distributed then surely theirs is the real authority?

The argument that power is based upon economic resources and that this power is legitimised by ideologies transmitted within the culture is

Figure 3.4 Women with dependent children, working full-time and part-time, Great Britain, 1979–81 and 1990–2

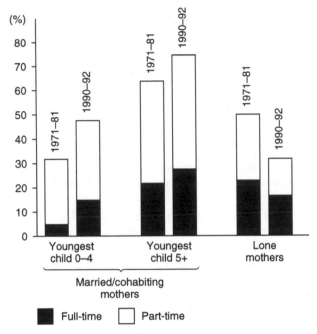

Sources: Adapted from International Year of the Family, *Fact Sheet 3*, Family Policies Unit.

one which to a degree, runs through most explanations. The male role within the family as the economic provider has been legitimised by social and occupational policies. The idea of the 'family wage' and the justification for paying men more than women was historically based upon the idea that all men had economic responsibilities which women did not. As we shall see in a later chapter, the role of the state was crucial in the institutionalisation in social legislation of the ideology of males as 'instrumental' financial providers and females as 'affective' care-providers within the family. So is male power within the family legitimised by a patriarchal culture and if so, what does this mean?

■ The family as ideology

The role of the family as an ideological model which has been instrumental in legitimising gender inequalities and constructing the nuclear family as the desired 'norm' for society, has been the focus of attention by many writers. In our language the word 'family' denotes both

Table 3.4 Divisions of household tasks, 1995

Task	How tasks should be shared*			Actual allocation of tasks		
	Mainly women	Mainly men	Shared equally	Mainly women	Mainly men	Shared equally
Organising household money and bills	14	17	66	40	31	28
Repairing household equipment	1	66	31	6	32	10
Household shopping	22	1	76	45	8	47
Doing household cleaning	36	1	62	68	4	27
Doing washing and ironing	58	–	40	84	3	12
Making evening meal	39	1	57	70	9	20
Doing evening dishes	11	11	75	33	28	37

* All respondents were asked; 'How should tasks be shared?'

Source: Adapted from Central Statistical Office, Focus on Women (HMSO, 1995); reproduced in Guardian (9 August 1995)

a specific form and a set of values. Advertisers use the phrase 'a family atmosphere' to suggest warmth and friendliness, a 'family entertainment' is one which is uncontroversial and pleasing, and we say someone was treated like 'one of the family'. The idea that 'the family' contains many people is illustrated by the way in which we use the word to describe a large size, for example a 'family home' is a house with a number of rooms, 'family-size' boxes of cornflakes and a 'family loaf' signifies that it is the largest one manufactured. In the popular culture, the lives of families are central to dramas, soap operas and situation comedies.

Women are essential to any definition of the family in our language and culture. We speak of a man as being a 'family man' and of a woman as being a 'career woman' because neither are 'naturally' in those spheres. We do not talk of a 'family woman' or a 'career man' because they already culturally exist in these occupations.

The modern construct of the Royal Family as characters in a soap opera, with 'good' and 'bad' women, 'strong' and 'weak' men, and led by a family matriarch is a powerful ideological image of gender roles. Within this cultural construction, it is concerns over 'family matters' such as imminent divorces, separations, engagements, marriages and pregnancies which dominate the popular press. The Royals are therefore 'de-politicised' and reinforce the gender stereotypes of women as mothers and men as public administrators or warriors. Richard Sennett's (1977) study of the cultural construct of the warm image of family life in the nineteenth century as a 'retreat' for men from the competitive world of commerce, shows that this was both a class and a gender ideological formation. Lower working-class family life was neither warm, comfortable or 'private' at this time, but the increasingly wealthy middle-classes were able to relate to the idea of the home as a place of sanctuary for men provided by women. This idea began to be adopted by the skilled respectable working class by the latter years of the nineteenth century and was reflected in trade union demands for the male to be paid a 'family wage' and for wives to stay at home, a new concept in working-class life (Gittins, 1985). As Sennett points out, the responsibility for the provision of the restorative powers of the home was that of the woman as the 'angel at the hearth'. He argues that this role in fact increased women's alienation and powerlessness. The argument that it is women who are seen as the providers of peace and tranquillity at home to their own cost (doing good – feeling bad) is echoed in social psychology (Brown and Harris, 1978).

Behind the ideology that 'a woman's place is in the home' and that home and family represent a haven for women from the dangers of the outside world are statistics on violence and abuse which contradict this cosy image. Women are in fact in more danger of rape, assault and death in the home and from spouses or partners than they are outside (see Figure 3.5).

There has recently been a great deal of media interest in the subject of domestic violence. In Scotland especially, the campaign of 'Zero Tolerance' which featured photographs on large advertising hoardings of beaten women, brought this issue into the public notice. The release from prison in 1995 of two women, Sara Thornton and Emma Humphreys, who had been found guilty of murdering violent partners and given mandatory life sentences further attracted media attention. How common is domestic violence? A survey carried out by Mooney (1993) in North London found that 27 per cent of women surveyed had experienced physical injury from partners, 37 per cent reported mental cruelty and 23 per cent reported rape. A study of women in refuges in England and Wales showed that almost 75 per cent had experienced prolonged violent assaults for the previous three or more years before seeking refuge (Pahl, 1995). Women in the ethnic minorities may experience greater difficulties in seeking help to escape from their violent situation because of cultural and 'community' pressures as well as the institutionalised racism of many statutory agencies (Mama, 1989). Despite the publicised cases of women who killed violent partners, the majority of people killed by domestic violence are women. In 1995 40–45 per cent of female homicide victims had been killed by present or former partners, but only 6 per cent of male victims had been killed by their partners (Home Office, 1995).

Norton *et al.* (1995) compared two different screening techniques for identifying women being subjected to domestic violence in their current

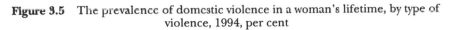

Figure 3.5   The prevalence of domestic violence in a woman's lifetime, by type of violence, 1994, per cent

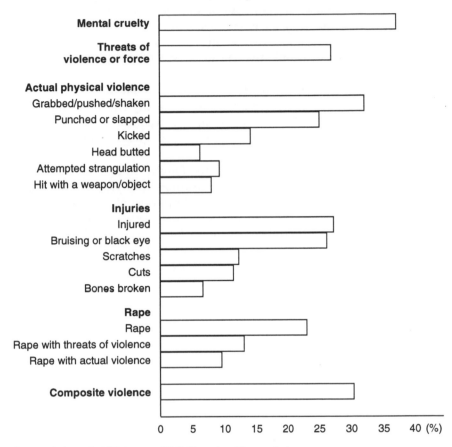

Sources: Independent (18 January 1994). Reproduced by permission.

pregnancy. The study was carried out in the USA and involved women with low obstetric risk and found that when they were asked simple and direct questions using an Abuse Assessment Screen, more violence against pregnant women was revealed (41 per cent using the assessment screen as compared with 14 per cent in the control group). Using the screen devised specifically to detect domestic violence, 15 per cent of women revealed violence in the last year. The personnel were trained in the administration of the screen and women were interviewed in private. The unit had also made arrangements to refer those women who needed and wanted help, to social workers or counsellors. Despite the high rates of domestic violence against pregnant women reported in this and other studies, such procedures are not widely used in the UK.

Nevertheless the importance of the family and their role within it is an integral part of most women's lives. Is this just the result of gender socialisation? or does a role within a family offer women a status and a function?

We have seen from social statistics that there is a great diversity of family forms and types, but they all point to the fact that the model of what constitutes 'the family' may have changed but there is still a desire on the part of the majority of people to form some type of grouping which could be referred to as 'a family'.

We began this chapter on 'the family' by stating that there was really no such thing, what we have in Britain today are many types of families. So when politicians talk of 'family values' and of 'traditional family life' it is rather difficult for a sociological approach to give credence to these appeals.

As we have seen however, models of 'the family' do have an ideological strength. Within this model of what constitutes the family, other forms such as lone parents, step-families and homosexual couples become marginalised and can be made to appear deviant. As we shall see in a later chapter, social policies on the family and social security benefits have been based upon a very restricted model of the family. Ideologies, then, do not just exist in people's imagination: they have a concrete and very real impact on people's lives.

■ Sociology and 'community'

Like 'the family' the phrase 'community' also has an important ideological function. Images of this type of community often appear to belong to the past, a past of rural villages and small populations where everyone knew everyone else. As with 'the family' the phrase 'community' belongs to a lost golden age, when it was 'safe to leave your door open' and ' everyone knew their neighbours'.

The most famous definition in sociology of this 'loss' of community was defined by Tonnies (1957). He distinguished between a pre-industrial society based upon *gemeinschaft*, a close-knit grouping of kinship networks; and the industrial society based upon *gesellschaft*, a loosely-based connection formed through associations and contacts. This formulation of a community as being based within a closely knit and largely pre-industrial value system and way of life tended to dominate much of sociological thinking in the early twentieth century. Many sociologists argued that urban and rural ways of life could be contrasted, with the urbanised society being far more loosely connected and potentially more alienating and dehumanising (Gans, 1967).

But was there ever this community or is this, too, a powerful ideology? Raymond Williams (1977) has argued that in our culture the country has become synonymous with ideas of goodness and purity and the town with ideas of evil and pollution. For Marxists, of course, it is the capitalist mode of production which is the basis of alienation and not urbanisation as such. Indeed, within Marxism there is a bias towards industrialisation and urbanism as being more advanced than rural or agricultural modes of production.

What do we mean when we talk of a community? It is a very ambiguous concept and Hillery (1955) actually calculated that there were sixty-four definitions available! But probably the most commonplace use of the phrase is in terms of a specific geographical location. The desire to move to the country from the town in order to 'live in a real community' is often articulated by (mostly middle class) people who obviously believe that a community is more likely to be found in a village than in a town. Sociological analyses of this ideological construction of 'the village in the mind' by Pahl (1965) have shown that this urban drift can be seen in terms of class conflicts between the middle-class incomers and the working-class villagers.

Studies of regions or areas are a fundamental part of community studies. These have often shown that a place may contain a specific population but this does not mean that it is a homogeneous one. Communities can be divided by class, status and ethnicity. Margaret Stacey's study of Banbury (1960), and others such as a study of a South Wales housing estate (Bell and Newby, 1971) and of other communities (Frankenburg 1965), and urban inner city areas (Rex and Moore, 1967) have all shown that just because people live in close proximity does not mean that they share other characteristics or that each community does not contain conflicts.

If we widen our definition of what constitutes 'a community' to include a social identity, then we look for groups of people who share a culture or other significant feature. We talk of 'ethnic communities', 'the elderly community' but again we are tending to view these as homogeneous. This is patently not the case: not all elderly people share the same characteristics, and an ethnic 'community' can include many hierarchies and power structures. The geographical placing of an ethnic group within a 'community' can conceal a form of institutionalised racism. Can we be certain that people of an ethnic group live in a certain place because they have the power to choose to do so, or are they forced to live in specific areas because of housing policies, fear of racial harassment and lack of equal opportunities? What of 'communities' of single mothers? Every large urban area will contain some housing estates with a predominant number of single women and children – is this also a 'community'?

We can see from these examples that some communities have actually been constructed by housing policies, but there has always been an element of the *social construction* of a community. The geographical location of industry has produced occupational communities based upon one type of work and exhibiting a *cultural community*. Mining communities were constructed in this way, based upon the fact that all the men worked in the same place and lived in close proximity to the pit. The culture which was built upon this occupational base is very familiar to us from literature, films, drama and documentaries and from sociological study (Dennis, Henriques and Slaughter, 1969), but in many ways it was a male-based culture. It stressed the masculine bonding of men in a dangerous occupation – men drank together in the pub, or working-men's club, sang in male voice choirs, played in brass bands, raced pigeons, followed rugby or football clubs: it was a male world. The female side of this well-documented 'community' culture is invisible. Women did not venture into the public male world of politics, trade unions or work; they lived in the community but were not a part of the public culture of it. This apparently close-knit cultural identity of a mining community, then, is a one-sided picture, women's lives were not a part of this public culture. They belonged to the hidden world of the family not the visible world of a cultural community.

But mining as an exclusively male job which created a male culture was an exception: most localities are not characterised by a single occupational group. Recent studies of inner-city deprived areas have shown that many 'communities' are today once again dominated by certain characteristics; the high number of people who are unemployed, single mothers or elderly women living alone. Beatrice Campbell (1993) in her studies of such communities argues that it is the women on these estates who represent 'the community'.

Hilary Graham (1987) also has argued that the idea of community life (as opposed to a culture) is an essentially feminine one. Women probably play more part in the construction of community life on a day-to-day basis. After all kinship and neighbour interaction is primarily through women. This is the basis of the feminist suspicion of the idea of placing 'care in the community'. For, they argue, this basically means that the caring role will be assigned to women within 'the family' rather than become the responsibility of a wider society (we return to an examination of the policy of Community Care in Chapter 6). In the provision of formal health and social care, too, community-based care is a predominantly female occupation. Health visitors, district nurses, home helps, 'community' midwives, are almost without exception, women (see Chapter 8).

Is the term 'community', then, just as ideological a concept as 'the family'? Both have been socially and historically constructed, both appear to be a definable unit and both carry models of form and content. But both have a diversity of forms and can be the site of gender, class and ethnic conflicts and inequalities.

To take a sociological approach to the study of both family and community is to attempt to define the structure and meaning given to these concepts within our society.

In this chapter, we have attempted to *deconstruct* the concepts of 'family' and 'community'. This is one of the strengths of a sociological approach, that it allows people to dissect certain taken-for-granted assumptions about everyday uses of familiar concepts. As we have seen, neither 'the family' or 'community' are straightforward and unambiguous concepts or structures. In Chapter 6 we look at the social policies which have played a part in institutionalising both these concepts and have constructed specific models of the family and of the role of the community.

■ The family, community and midwifery care

In the case histories that follow it can be seen that midwives come into contact with many different types of families. The role of the midwife should be different in different settings and always be responsive to the individual needs of the woman and her partner. There is a danger in stereotyping women and their families and slotting individuals into categories based on a superficial judgement of their social class, status, family type and position. Stereotyping is a straitjacket to good care. It is easy to assume that the unmarried mother needs more support and advice or guidance on diet, screening tests, and smoking just because she is not married. It is also easy to assume that because a woman is married and appears content, that all is well.

Case Study 3.1   'Adjusting to pregnancy'

Mrs Ali is an Asian woman who first arrives at the Antenatal Clinic when she is twenty weeks pregnant. She is wearing a traditional Muslim dress. The records and letter from her GP indicate that this is her first pregnancy. She is not accompanied by her husband or by a female relative. The clinic receptionist has already filled in some details on the booking-clinic sheet and has assumed Mrs Ali is married. Mrs Ali sits away from the other women waiting in the clinic; the midwife notices that she stares at the floor and sighs. The midwife stands in front of Mrs Ali and opens the conversation by asking, 'Do you speak English?' Mrs Ali sighs and complains about racism in the health service. The midwife then invites Mrs Ali to join her in a small room. The midwife sits behind the desk and in silence puts the papers in order. During the course of the booking clinic interview it transpires that Mrs Ali is a solicitor and is aged 36 years. Eventually the midwife manages to put aside her preconceived ideas and prejudices and begins to communicate in a more effective way. As the rapport between them improves Mrs Ali describes some of her feelings. She eventually explains that she is experiencing great difficulty in adjusting to her pregnancy and fears the loss of her status, position, income and independence. She has not contemplated termination of pregnancy but appears depressed and withdrawn. She does not want to discuss ways in which her care can be organised, the place of birth or aspects such as her medical history and diet. She looks pale and tired.

The midwife begins to notice Mrs Ali apparent depression. She closes the door of the office and unplugs the telephone. She sits alongside her, asks some gentle questions and begins to listen carefully to Mrs Ali's verbal and non-verbal communication. Eventually Mrs Ali begins to trust the midwife. It also transpires that she lives with her husband, who works away for much of the time and with her parents-in-law who are devout Muslims. They live in a very large house in a run-down area of the city. Sharing the house are an uncle, a nephew and a cousin. She eventually explains that she did not intend becoming pregnant and does not want to be pregnant at all. She explains that she resents what she calls 'the intrusion of her body' but immediately feels guilty for saying this. She says that her husband and extended family have insisted that she continues with her pregnancy and leaves her job once the baby is born. There have been some discussions about her mother-in-law caring for the baby but Mrs Ali feels that this may not be for the best. There are no child-care facilities at her work and she has not considered either a child-minder or a nanny. Her husband is frequently angry about her response to the pregnancy and has resorted to physical violence against her in the last few months.

■ Questions and discussion points

- How does Mrs Ali's family structure compare with traditional images of the family?
- Would you expect Mrs Ali to have the problems that are described in the case study?, If not why not?
- Are there any other significant aspects of Mrs Ali's pregnancy?
- When the midwife asks Mrs Ali if she speaks English is this reasonable or are her actions based on a stereotypical image of Asian women in the country?
- Are there any ways in which the midwife can alter the balance of power described in this encounter?
- How can the midwife help Mrs Ali in adjusting to this pregnancy?
- How can a deeper understanding of the family, marriage, ethnicity and power help the midwife to offer more sensitive care?
- How does Mrs Ali's family differ from the imaginary 'typical family'?
- Mrs Ali eventually revealed that she had been subjected to domestic violence. How should the midwife respond and what would be appropriate referral policies?

Case Study 3.2   A family group

Mrs Jones calls at her GP's surgery with her 15 year old daughter Janette. Mrs Jones is 35 years old, divorced and ten weeks pregnant. She admits that she is not sure who the father of her child is but thinks it is probably Geoff who is a long-distance lorry-driver. She has had a relationship with him for some years but they do not intend to marry. Geoff lives some distance away in another town but often stays the night. Mrs Jones smokes heavily, drinks socially and has asthma. She has had four pregnancies which have variously resulted in a termination of pregnancy when she was 16, a miscarriage and two live births. She is underweight and very breathless as she enters the waiting room. She lives on Social Security benefits and earnings from her part-time job as a cleaner.

Janette, her daughter, is 15 and pregnant. She has a steady boyfriend called Mike. She lives at home with her mother and her older brother called John. Mike, her boyfriend does not get on well with his parents and has been sleeping on the sofa at Janette's house for some months. They do not intend to marry but when both babies are born they believe that they will be able to find other accommodation. Mike is just 17 and unemployed.

Janette is physically fit and well. She is excited about having a child of her own and a new baby brother or sister. She is worried about her mother's health and how her smoking will affect both babies.

The family group consists of Mrs Jones, sometimes Geoff, Janette, her boyfriend Mike and John, Janette's brother.

■ Questions and discussion points

- Do you think that Janette lives in a supportive family?
- Using Functionalist theories of the family comment on how this family functions as a social process.
- Describe how this family can be seen in relation to society as a whole. Does it conform to the ideology of the family?
- On the basis of your experience as a midwife does the typical family exist?
- As the midwife who meets Mrs Jones and her daughter for the first time, what aspects of their care would you consider first?
- What immediate advice could you offer this family?
- How can learning about families help midwives to give better care?

Key points

- There is not one model of the family but many different formations.
- The traditional family is a social construction symbolising the British norm.
- It is difficult to compare families over time and make assumptions about the relative strengths and weaknesses of 'the family'.
- Ethnicity as well as social class are significant variables in the analysis of families.
- Sociological theories of the family include Functionalist and Feminist. Functionalists are concerned with the function of the family in relation to society as a whole and feminists are concerned with internal workings and roles within families.
- Feminist studies of families look carefully at gender roles, treatment and attitudes towards children, and the basis of power and authority within the family.
- The ideology or images of 'the family' help to perpetuate myths and half truths.

- Marriage is less popular than previously, divorce rates are increasing but there is still a trend towards the setting up of 'family groups'.
- Community like family is an ambiguous concept.
- Beware of stereotyping women and their families. Good care must be sensitive, thoughtful and non judgmental.
- Care must be based on the needs of individuals and needs change as society changes. For example, women undertaking paid work outside the home have different needs to women who do unpaid work in the home.
- Single does not necessarily mean unsupported.
- Midwives should try to understand the different roles and responsibilities women have in different households and offer care and advice that is appropriate in that particular context.

Chapter 4

Social aspects of pregnancy and childbirth

A sociological approach to pregnancy and childbirth centralises the social aspect of these physiological and biological events. Sociologists emphasise the impact of society's values, beliefs and patterns of behaviour on the way in which they are interpreted and given meaning by people. Pregnancy and childbirth are social events in that they take place within a surrounding economic and social system and are understood within a cultural value system. Like other social events, such as marriage and death, interpretations and meanings given by a society are subject to historical change and will also exhibit social class and ethnic variations. What singles out pregnancy and childbirth from other social events however, is the exclusively gendered nature of the experience. No other life event is exclusively a matter for one sex only. Even a previously predominantly (never exclusive) male experience such as active service and death in war has, during this century, become a civilian experience shared by women and children. Even traditional male occupations such as mining, deep-sea fishing or oil-rig working have been undertaken by women at certain times: male predominance is due more to social and organisational policies and ideologies than to biological determination. But pregnancy and childbirth 'belong' to women. This explains why feminist scholarship has virtually monopolised sociological and historical analyses of the social construction of pregnancy and birth. A common thread which runs through all accounts is that of the domination of a patriarchal culture which first appropriated, then controlled and organised, this female experience. The sociological approach, then, is to stress the nature of power relations in society and how these affect the ways in which pregnancy and childbirth are experienced. In order to illustrate the social aspect of the interpretation of this experience, we can look back historically to see how the social meaning placed upon pregnancy and childbirth has changed historically.

■ The private event

The overwhelmingly obvious change in the social experience of pregnancy and childbirth has been the move from the essentially private nature of the event to its public recognition over the past century. Michel

Foucault (1980) has argued that prior to the nineteenth century, society was far more open and outspoken in its public recognition of sexual activity and childbirth, but Victorian society whilst in many ways obsessed by sex (covering up the legs of pianos for example), also sought to organise and control sexual activity within the heterosexual family group. All matters relating to sex, especially for women, became areas of secrecy and guilt. Sex became a powerful discourse through which other activities were also controlled. Laws governing the practice of male homosexuality also became a part of British society for the first time in the nineteenth century, as the famous trial of Oscar Wilde was to illustrate.

A woman's social reputation became founded upon her sexual activity (or rather lack of it). The 'ideal' woman was to be sexually attractive but sexually inactive, at least until marriage, and even then it was often considered to be desirable for a woman to appear sexually uninterested as a mark of her 'ladylike' nature. This obviously placed a great deal of restriction upon women's lives and led to women observing and policing their own behaviour and that of their daughters. This is the main point of the Foucault (1977) analysis of the control of the population in a modern society, that surveillance moves from the control of others and that individuals actually begin to police their own behaviour as they feel constantly under observation.

Pregnancy, which once had been celebrated in classical art as the pinnacle of womanhood, now became a shameful condition which was never mentioned in polite company. Women's clothes changed from the 'Empire line' of the late eighteenth century and the Regency period, which exaggerated a pregnant look, to clothes which were designed to conceal this 'interesting condition'. It must be remembered that for most women until the twentieth century, pregnancy was a semi-permanent state. Working-class and even middle-class women could not afford to buy clothes which would only be wearable during the short period when they were not pregnant and so the concealment factor was an important one. But although pregnancy was much more common than it is today, it was often viewed as 'shameful' as it was a public illustration of female sexual activity. In a culture which defined women as either 'pure' or 'fallen', pregnancy was the proof that both 'types' of women had engaged in the same act. The emphasis on the legitimacy or otherwise, of the child was the point of differentiation between 'madonna' and 'whore' but pregnancy as an event was common to both.

The definition of childbirth as an event in the private sphere can be interpreted in two ways:

1. the way in which childbirth was culturally viewed as a private 'secret' known only to women;
2. the actual site of childbirth which until the 1930s took place predominantly in the private space of the home.

Childbirth was an area of myth, secrecy, terror and potential death. The 'natural' aspect of it did not change the fact that for many women it was an event to be dreaded and feared even if children were desired. Generations of women grew up surrounded by tales of pain and horror which were made all the more potent because of their secrecy and female exclusivity. We will see in Chapter 8 how this image of secrecy and guilt attached itself to the occupation of midwife and to midwifery as a practice. There were, of course differences in the way in which childbirth was experienced by the wealthy in contrast to the working classes. For the rich, and especially the monarchy, childbirth was always more of a 'public' event. Royal births had to be witnessed by appointed courtiers to make certain of the legitimacy of the newborn child as heir. In wealthy families too, the event was of great economic importance as it was concerned with the ownership of property. In this way, childbirth was of a primarily social and economic significance, – it was the child as a means of legitimising the transference of wealth rather than as an individual being. This may also explain the differences in historical patterns of 'mothering' between the social classes. However, for most working-class women who were crammed into the overcrowded slums and back-to-back housing of the industrial towns or the damp cottage hovels in villages, privacy was also non-existent. Women gave birth on straw pallets on floors of rooms occupied by whole families or in a bed which was shared by others. Therefore, the actual event of childbirth was lacking in either privacy or comfort, but the myths and interpretations surrounding it relegated it to the area of guilt and secrecy. Women were ignorant about the workings of their bodies as reminiscences show (Humphries and Gordon, 1993), sex education did not exist and documentary images of childbirth were not shown until the mid-1940s.

■ The public event

In the past few years, popular culture has 'rediscovered' the beauty of pregnancy. Now that pregnancy is an increasingly rare event in women's lives, it is much more celebrated and pictured. Special maternity clothes which first became available to the wealthy who were pregnant less often, were produced for the masses in the post-war period. Originally, these clothes were dull and consisted of a smock which continued the covering-up function. However by the 1960s, fashionable clothes for pregnant women were sold in every high street and shops specialising in them were created. A whole new area of fashion opened up to cater for this changed interpretation of pregnancy. This was at a time when attitudes to sex were changing and a whole new popular culture emphasising sexual liberation and increased female freedom was constructed. By the 1980s, female celebrities appeared on television and openly discussed their pregnancy and were photographed in close-up. Pregnancy was no longer viewed as shameful, but remnants of traditional attitudes remain, for the nude photo of a pregnant Demi Moore on the front cover of *Vanity Fair* magazine was still considered to be controversial as recently as 1992. How can sociology explain this pattern of the 'normalisation' of pregnancy in our culture? Is it because as a rarer occurrence it now has a higher status and is it connected with the increasingly public role that women now occupy in society? Both these explanations may be valid, but what is evident is that a changing economic structure with a greater female participation in the workforce and a changed cultural discourse have contributed to a new social construct of the meaning of pregnancy. To be pregnant in the 1990s is not the same social experience as being pregnant in previous decades. A whole new range of meanings and interpretations are now in place which did not exist previously.

■ The scan – 'seeing' the baby

The development of ultrasound scanning in obstetrics has been the subject of much feminist and sociological interest. Its now almost total use on all women as part of the normal monitoring process during pregnancy has not been without its critics. Pressure groups have consistently argued against its routine use but now the criticisms are from within the medical establishment. The organisation AIMS (Association for Improvement in Maternity Services) has criticised its routine use on all women and has called for more research into effects (Squire, 1984). A radiologist, Margaret Furness (1987) has also been critical of its use and of the chances of misdiagnosis and error which insufficient training can produce. In 1993 a special issue of the *AIMS Journal* continued the campaign against the routine use of ultrasound in pregnancy. Green and Stalham (1993) in their review of antenatal screening techniques comment on how extraordinary it is that scanning is so widely used when so little is known about its long-term effects. Dowswell and Hewison (1994) are equally concerned and argue that as yet little is known about the possible positive or negative effects of early scans. They argue that routine use has been adopted without the fundamental questions of safety and efficacy being answered. They recommend large controlled trials but fail to consider the difficulties associated with defining a control group willing to forgo a procedure now considered an essential stage in becoming a mother. The tide may yet turn.

Interestingly, the actual division of labour which accompanies operating the scan is illustrative of the domination of medicine over other paramedical occupations. Radiographers actually operate the scan but it is up to doctors to interpret the result. The lack of communication between operators and pregnant women has also been a cause for concern.

Women reported to a NCT (National Childbirth Trust) survey in 1984 on the lack of attention and information given to them by operators. Some women reported the way in which they felt pushed to the periphery of attention as doctors concentrated solely on the image on the screen and ignored them (Price, 1990, p. 139).

Writers such as Petchesky (1987), have analysed the use of the scan from a feminist perspective. She argues that the development of fetal images is a part of the technological masculine-based culture which has pervaded all aspects of maternity care. The technique of ultra-scanning was developed during the war as a weapon of detection in submarine warfare and then transferred to obstetrics, first in the USA and then, later, in Britain by the late 1960s. Petchesky (1987) argues that it coincided with the fall in the birth rate and the need for obstetricians to look for 'new fields' of professional practice and control.

But it is its ability to lay bare what has always previously been hidden which interests sociologists most. Its application has been to make 'public' and visual that which was 'private' and hidden. The 'inside' and 'outside' of a woman's body have become merged and indistinguishable. From a Foucauldian point of view, it has increased the degree of control and surveillance possible and also enabled women to view themselves. The increased interest in the fetus by medical practitioners has led some writers (Hubbard, 1985) to argue that it is being seen as a 'mini-patient' and an autonomous being with needs separate from that of the mother.

But 'seeing the baby on the scan' is almost universally popular with women and it must be remembered that many technological developments in childbirth have been demanded by women themselves (Lewis, 1980; Hunt and Symonds, 1995). Having a scan is now eagerly anticipated by most women as their chance to see the baby and know that 'everything is all right'. This could be viewed as an alternative interpretation of its use, that women themselves have appropriated it and have turned it into a part of a female world of the family and the keeping of memories in terms of photographs. It is now quite common for prospective grandparents to be presented with a photo of their unborn grandchild. Sometimes when the sex of the child is revealed, the photo is contained on a card which is 'signed' by 'Joshua' or 'Amy'. But how can we understand this phenomenon? To any other age but our own this would be totally inexplicable behaviour. Try explaining to someone from another culture that you have received a communication from a person who is not yet born! This would appear to belong to a world of magic and supernatural happenings, not from a scientific and rational society.

A sociological 'reading' of the technological development of scanning technique would encompass a placing of its operation within the masculinised culture and also the professional and occupational hierarchies. But there are two alternative interpretations possible. One is that it is yet another example of the 'male take-over' of aspects of reproduction and the other that women themselves have appropriated elements of the technology in order to gain a measure of control. But the visibility of the fetus has also led to a redefinition of the responsibilities of the pregnant woman. Now that progress can be monitored, it is increasingly stressed that women have a measure of individual responsibility to adopt healthy behavioural patterns in order to produce a 'perfect' baby. The most focused-upon area of 'health risk' behaviour among women has been that of smoking during pregnancy.

■ Smoking, pregnancy and social class

The one health education message that any woman attending for antenatal checks cannot fail to have received is that of the dangers posed to her unborn child by her smoking. The message is constant and unrelenting in its target: women who smoke are showing a degree of irresponsibility and are ignoring medical advice. Smoking is often given as the cause of low birthweight babies. Sociologists are very suspicious of a single causal factor analysis as they would wish to broaden the argument and look instead for connections but not necessarily causes. This analysis can be applied to smoking and low birthweight babies, one vital factor which is missing from this simple equation smoking = low birthweight is that of social class and all the attendant disadvantages that can mean.

As Oakley has chronicled (1989) many writers have noted the connection between smoking in pregnancy, low birthweight and other variables such as later development in reading, height and weight by the age of 7 and even the gaining of educational qualifications in adult life. In other words, since 1969, when this concern was first recorded (Butler and Alberman, 1969), mothers who smoke when pregnant can be 'blamed' for most adverse circumstances that affect their children into adulthood. But is smoking just a useful peg on which to hang the blame for other social circumstances such as low social support, stress and worry and depression, all of which can be said to stem from social and economic deprivation? Smoking throughout the general population is inversely related to indices of affluence. This means that smokers are most likely to be tenants not home-owners, not to own a car or a telephone and not to have good housing standards such as central heating (Oakley, 1989). Interestingly in a study by Brooke *et al.* (1989) the authors set out to investigate the effects of smoking, alcohol, caffeine consumption, socio-economic factors and psychological stress on birthweight. The sample was 1513 women. They found that smoking was the most important single factor and concluded that social and psychological factors had little or no direct effect on birthweight corrected for gestational age. They argued that only four of their socio-economic and stress factors significantly reduced birthweight and these effects became non-significant after making allowance for smoking. To assume a simple cause and effect would be naive. The real question is 'why is smoking more prevalent among poorer women than middle-class women? It must be stressed that a socio-cultural activity such as smoking is a product of social structures such as poverty.

Smoking among women has declined much more slowly than among men, and teenage girls are more likely than their male counterparts to smoke. Despite this, pregnant women are told that it is their 'duty' to give up for the sake of the baby. But this advice does not take into account the surrounding circumstances of a woman's life which have probably encouraged her to smoke in the first place. Hilary Graham (1987) has shown that most pregnant women have received and understood all the health education messages and yet many continue to smoke. Why?

As Hilary Graham's study shows, smoking for many women who are living under great stress and worry is a coping mechanism, in her study of low-income families over 28 per cent of mothers said that it was the way in which they managed their everyday lives.

Ann Oakley's study of women who smoke during pregnancy (1989) also uncovered two other reasons; a low birthweight baby was seen as quite desirable and not necessarily to be prevented; and medical advice was simply either not believed, or defied. As one of her respondents said, '[My sister-in-law] already had one boy at 9lb near enough, and she didn't want a big baby, she wanted a small baby, that was the reason she smoked!' (Oakley , 1989, p. 326).

The defiance of medical and organisational control can be witnessed every time you pass the entrance to a maternity unit in any hospital, anywhere. The entrance is strewn with cigarette ends and there is always a number of women who, despite the weather, congregate outside the hospital to smoke. It could be argued that medical technology itself can be seen as the reason why low birthweight babies are not seen as a problem. After all special care baby units are constantly being portrayed as being able to keep alive very premature babies and this could be factor in the seemingly low priority given by some women to the low birthweight of babies.

As Oakley argues, the problem with the individualistic health education model is that it fails to locate smoking within the other structures of many women's lives. Poverty, bad housing, unemployment, depression and low social support are all factors in producing not just a tendency to smoke but also lower standards of health generally (see Chapter 2).

The increased public nature of pregnancy has, of course paralleled the now public nature of childbirth itself. The actual event of childbirth was always shrouded in mystery. Unlike pregnancy there have been very few actual depictions of it in art. The icon of the madonna and child which has dominated European art since the Renaissance has always portrayed a very sanitised picture of mother and newly born baby. The pictorial depiction of childbirth itself did not occur until female artists such as

Frida Kahlo broke through the male-dominated form in the mid-twentieth century. Likewise in novels and drama, the act of childbirth was an 'off-stage' occurrence. Men, of course, were never present at childbirth and so were always depicted as pacing up and down outside the room. The absence of men from birth until the 1970s as compared with the situation today is discussed further in the following chapter.

Women often mysteriously died whilst giving birth but the description of the actual event (like male deaths in battle) was absent. This 'absence' of a cultural recognition was also evident in the forms of popular culture of the twentieth century. It was not until the late 1930s in the film, *Gone With The Wind,* that a childbirth scene was shown and this was censored by some local authorities as too 'horrific'. By the end of the Second World War, childbirth was the subject of documentaries which were part of the post-war cultural placing of it within the new health service. The popular magazine *Picture Post* also carried photos of childbirth in this period. This trend continued, and by the 1990s childbirth scenes which were far more graphic than those shown forty years previously, were a part of family viewing in popular television programmes. What this change has meant is that for the first time in centuries, women now see their private experience as part of the public sphere. This changed meaning and interpretation has meant that both pregnancy and childbirth are now in the public domain of a shared culture.

Understandably, this cultural transition has attracted many sociological and historical analyses and has become a focus for feminist scholarship. The change in the social meaning of childbirth from an event in the private female sphere to the public sphere has been analysed in terms of a struggle in the social relations of power and authority. The analysis which has dominated this study of the changing site and nature of childbirth has been that of a feminist school of writing which has placed patriarchal power as the motivating force. The place of fathers and men in birth is discussed in Chapter 5.

■ Hospitalisation and the male 'takeover'

The most important factor in the changed cultural meaning of childbirth has been the change in site from the private sphere of the home to the public sphere of the hospital. This represents the greatest change in the experience of childbirth. How, when and why did this happen ?

There were many intersecting motivations of the state, political parties and professional groups which surrounded this move. But first, the move itself, when did it begin to take place in the public sphere?

The steady increase in hospital birth began before the Second World War and gained in momentum in the affluent post-war period of the 1960s and 1970s until by the 1990s it is almost the universal experience.

This medicalisation of childbirth has been defined by a powerful school of feminist theory as the expression of patriarchal power. Writers such as Donnison (1988) and Oakley (1986) argued forcibly that this move meant the subjection of women to male power and of the decline in authority and status of the female midwife to the role of maternity nurse to the male obstetrician. This view, epitomised in many ways by the wide ranging work of Anne Oakley firmly places patriarchy as the power structure within which childbirth has lost its place as the female power base (Oakley, 1986). Oakley sees the move of pregnancy and childbirth into the male-dominated sphere of medicine as one which has robbed women of autonomy and control over their bodies. Studies of the treatment of women by masculinised medical philosophy and practice (Martin, 1989; Moscucci, 1990; Ehrenreich and English, 1973) have rightly become central to a feminist critique of the supposedly 'objective' nature of medicine.

Many of the arguments which accompanied the transition from home birth to hospital, can effectively be analysed in terms of a dominant patriarchal structure. But to acknowledge that the predominantly male professions gained from the hospitalisation of birth, is not in itself an explanation of *why* this change took place.

There were (and still remain) two primary reasons for the move to hospital and the two are very much connected; safety and the desire for pain relief.

The relatively high levels of maternal mortality in the 1930s prompted political and professional demands for increased safety in childbirth. These demands were increasingly echoed by many women themselves who perceived hospital as somehow 'safer'. It has consistently been shown, however, that births which were attended by midwives carried less risk than those in hospital (Tew, 1995). Also, the likelihood of maternal mortality, unlike other fatalities, did not have a social-class correlation. Women from the upper social classes (who had the services of a doctor and a private nursing home) were, relatively, more 'at risk' than those of the working classes who had a home birth attended by a midwife. The risk of infection was probably greater in a hospital than in even poor standards of housing. Nevertheless, hospitalisation became perceived as the preferred safe option and even today that is the prime reason given by many women when asked about their choice between hospital or home. First, it has to be remembered that post-war hospitals became vastly more stringent in their hygiene practices, antibiotics were discovered and infection virtually disappeared. But even when they were not so 'safe' from infection, hospital births were gaining in popular esteem as letters to the midwifery press in the 1930s bear out (Hunt and Symonds, 1995). Changes in the pre-war organisation and status of hospitals and the lessening of costs helped the process. But if there was no validity in the claim that hospital was safer how and why did it become a commonplace belief amongst the majority of women?

Certainly the socialisation process has played a part in this – the vast majority of children today are born to mothers who themselves were born in hospital. Over the past three generations it has now become the cultural 'norm' and so any challenge to this will now appear to be a radical one. Older women who had their babies at home are in a minority and may not have had a very positive experience to relate.

Hospitals have also changed their image and meaning in society. Historically, they were seen as dark and forbidding institutions and connected with connotations of pauperism and death (Granshaw and Porter, 1990). This view has changed dramatically this century, the less stigmatising approach of Local Authority hospitals in the inter-war years and the post-war expansion of modern hospital buildings have contributed to this changed meaning. They play a large role in the popular culture too: dramas and television soap operas are set in hospitals with the medical and nursing staff portrayed as the heroes and heroines. But this portrayal only *reflects* the cultural change rather than creating it.

Hospitalisation was part of a scientifically based modernist culture which dominated in the USA and in Britain in the post-war years. They represented the bright new sanitised world of medical science triumphant. In this modern world, pain began to appear as a throwback to the dark ages. In other fields of health-care provision, noticeably dentistry, techniques to lessen pain were given top priority.

During the 1930s there was a growing demand that childbirth should be rendered as painless as possible. In America, the technique known as 'twilight sleep' became available and was given publicity. In Britain, the access to analgesics and anaesthetics had a distinctive social-class correlation. The RCM had noted this inequality in 1934 and in 1947, the report by the Royal Commission on Population calculated that 3 out of 5 women from the professional classes received analgesics compared with only 1 in 5 of manual working class women (Hunt and Symonds, 1995). The main reason why richer women could buy themselves a measure of pain relief was due to two factors: increased availability of anaesthetics in nursing homes and private hospitals; and the appropriation of these techniques and technology by the medical profession. Midwives were not allowed to administer chloroform or any anaesthetic without the presence of a doctor. After 1934, they were allowed to use the gas-and-air Minnit machine (with another midwife present) but this was so heavy and cumbersome to carry that it mitigated against widespread use especially in rural areas.

During this time, there was another interesting trend in the battle against pain in childbirth, the intellectual reinforcement of childbirth as a 'natural' phenomenon. The government report of 1937 actually blamed women themselves for their 'increased sensibility to pain' (Ministry of Health, 1937). The obstetrician Grantley Dick-Read (1950, 1951) first argued that childbirth was as much a psychological experience as a physical one, and achieved a large following for his technique of 'natural' childbirth. The 'mind over matter' school of thought did attract followers but most of these books (as with similar books today) were bought and read by a predominantly educated middle class (we will examine further the social-class composition of the movements for natural childbirth in Chapter 8). For the majority of working-class women however, the move to hospital for the birth became an increasingly sought-after option for many reasons, its perceived 'safety', as well as families' own bad housing conditions.

The *technology* of pain relief became centred within the hospital. As kitchen table operations to remove tonsils and appendix became obsolete so too did home births. The placing of this technology in hospitals was not, however, a random accident, it was a conscious *social decision*.

Within sociology, especially in America, there is a school of thought which focuses exclusively upon the role of technology in social and economic change (Kerr *et al.*, 1973; Blauner, 1964). In this view, technology acts as an autonomous social agent which constructs people's work and leisure patterns of behaviour. It is almost as though it exists in a super-natural way completely separate from any human influence or ownership. This view would be rejected by both Marxist and many feminist writers. Marxists argue that technology is only a part of the ownership of the means of production in a society and therefore its implementation must be in the interests of the ruling class (Braverman, 1974). Feminists would point to the gender relationship inherent in the use of technology (Cockburn, 1990). Technology, it is argued, has been appropriated within a patriarchal culture by men as an instrument of power which excludes women as users but positions them in the role of passive recipients. When looking at the increased use of technology in childbirth we can see many of these patterns at work. As Ruth Schwarz-Cowan (1989) has argued, 'tools are not passive instruments confined to doing our bidding, but have a life of their own. People use tools to do work, but tools also define and constrain the ways in which it is possible and likely that people will behave' (Schwarz-Cowan, 1989, p. 9).

■ The medicalisation of birth

It is important to state at the outset that the medicalisation of birth and obstetric practice that is firmly based on the medical model of care is not all bad. The medical model tends to assume that the human body, pregnant or not, is basically a machine. Machines have individual components which periodically malfunction and need intervention and repair. Where midwives have been happy to watch and wait for the whole body effectively to bring forth a healthy infant, the medical model almost compels the medical man to intervene because he is present. This mechanistic view of the woman produces language such as dysfunctional labour, uterine inertia, incoordinate uterine action and the mechanism of labour. The woman experiencing childbirth tends to be viewed as a series of components on a production line (Hunt and Symonds, 1995) and not as a whole person whose psychological needs interact with her physical and emotional needs.

However, many lives have been saved by medical interventions and many woman have desperately wanted, and achieved, pain-free labours. Many women (probably the majority in the 1990s) have agreed to, or asked for, effective pain relief in labour. Techniques in obstetric analgesia and anaesthesia have developed rapidly in response to what women want.

It is also true to say that birth in hospital has increased from 61.3 per cent in 1960 to 96.87 per cent in 1992 (OPCS). This move from home to hospital was associated with a corresponding fall in the perinatal mortality rate and naturally associated with safety. However, Tew (1995) and Campbell and Macfarlane (1995) have consistently demonstrated a basic error of deduction in assuming that a causal relationship existed between these two related statistics.

But to suggest that women went to hospital just for pain relief is, as we have seen, an over-simplification. Many will argue that the pain of birth only becomes intolerable when a women is in hospital, removed from her own environment and where her ability to exert control over the events is lost. Arney (1982) argues that pain relief is in itself a way of exerting control over women. An epidural renders a woman powerless, and immobile in more ways than one. O'Connor (1995) writing about home birth in Ireland argues that the pain of humiliation whether sexual or otherwise is part of the pain of childbirth but this is never recognised by obstetricians. She argues that obstetricians themselves have created the need for epidurals by introducing such practices as amniotomy, active birth regimes and syntocinon. She believes that when women are taken to hospital, confined to bed and catheterised and where this leads to an increase in operative delivery then the need for greater and greater pain relief is apparent. The view is supported by Sally Inch and explained in her theory of the assumption of pathology and the cascade of intervention (Inch, 1989, p. 244).

But there is far more to this change in birth than either, on the woman's part, a desire for pain relief or, on the hospital side, the male takeover of birth. It is true that for many years skills that were unique to women and generally based in the home have been eroded by the new professionals. The natural knowledge of women, their opinions and experience are devalued by the so-called experts. The acquired knowledge of the professional women (the midwife) it seems, has to dominate the experiential knowledge of the natural woman (Hunt and Symonds, 1995). As a result women have often lost confidence in their ability to give birth unaided. The culture of dependency ensures that the really important decisions in life are made by the doctor who is always the expert. So birth bccamc pathology, an abnormal state and an illness requiring diagnosis and medical intervention to ensure a safe outcome. As Ivan Illich (1976) so clearly explains, 'Diagnosis always intensifies stress, defines incapacity, imposes inactivity, and focuses apprehension on non-recovery, on uncertainty, and on one's dependence on future medical findings, all of which amounts to a loss of autonomy or self definition.'

Birth in hospital led to a dramatic increase in medical intervention in birth and a corresponding reduction in the midwives' autonomy, skill and activity in birth (Robinson, 1989). Indeed as birth became more likely to be defined as abnormal and potentially dangerous so the need for intervention, medical expertise and technological intervention grew. The adage of 'only normal in retrospect' (Percival, 1970; Schwarz, 1990) rapidly became part of conventional wisdom. It was only the foolish, the wayward and the highly strung who would risk embarking on this hazardous process without medical guidance and technological inter- vention. It may surprise some women to know that a positive outcome of a healthy mother and healthy baby can be achieved without scans, induction, epidural analgesia and forceps delivery but this is now outside most women's experience.

Many of the changes in the management of normal labour stem from the contribution made by an Irish obstetrician, O'Driscoll, who together with Meagher (1986) developed a system of 'active management of labour'. These authors, who incidentally describe midwives as nurses, believed that a labour should never last longer than twelve hours. They developed a protocol for dealing with a newly defined abnormality of 'prolonged labour' which required interventions such as artificial rupture of the membranes, augmentation using syntocinon, frequent vaginal examinations, electronic fetal monitoring, restriction in movement (the woman is confined to bed), more analgesia because the contractions are more painful and often some form of surgical delivery. The cascade of intervention described by MacLennan (1978) was an inevitable con- sequence. O'Driscoll and Meagher claimed that their intervention regime reduced the numbers of operative deliveries but their work fails to measure the psychological effects of intervention and the longer-term physical and psychological pathology.

As long ago as 1973 Ian Kennedy described the 'technological imperative'. He argued that in the technological revolution there is an urgency to master new techniques. As technology develops so does the desire to make use of it. He calls for more thought and asks for consideration of costs and benefits. It is important to consider that just because 'we can', it does not mean that 'we must' on every occasion.

As discussed earlier in this chapter, ultrasonic scanning is another example of the 'technological imperative'. According to Enkin *et al.* (1995), 'Whether ultra-sound imaging should be used routinely for prenatal screening or used selectively for specific interventions has not, as yet, been firmly established' (p. 40). Yet the ultrasonic scan is now an established part of normal antenatal care for all women. Antenatal care is conducted in hospitals where the expensive machinery is stored and must be used frequently to justify the capital cost.

In September 1994 Michel Odent launched a 'campaign for Eliminating the Nocebo Effect of Prenatal Care'. He describes the 'Nocebo Effect' as 'when a doctor or anyone else does more harm than good by interfering with someone's fantasy life, imagination or beliefs'. He argues against prenatal care that focuses on potential problems and believes that it has a negative effect on the well-being of pregnant women. He argues that care will be much better when the word 'routine' is excluded from the vocabulary of obstetricians and midwives. In the litigation-conscious USA the caesarian section rate is now 1:4. It is a comparatively safe and painless operation, women seem to want it and obstetricians have the technology, the takeover of birth is almost complete.

But the story does not end here. We shall read how in the 1990s social policy in Britain has shifted away from hospitals, from medical intervention and towards care in the community. The dripping tap has continued to drip and through documents such as 'Having a Baby in Europe'(1985), 'The Vision' (1986), RCM, 'Towards a Healthy Nation'(1987), The Social Services Committee Report (1992) and finally 'Changing Childbirth' (DOH, 1993), a model of care based on health rather than illness is emerging. The cynic may argue that the motivation may be financial rather than any deep concern for women's experience of childbirth but the end result has the potential to undo some of the harm caused by the medicalisation of birth. It may well depend on the ability of midwives to rise to the challenge.

■ Birth as a social experience

We have seen how the meaning of both pregnancy and childbirth has changed historically within society. At all times though there has never been a universal experience of either. This experience has been mediated through the social structures of social class and ethnicity. We have seen, for instance, that the pre-war maternal mortality rates had social class connotations, with the middle classes having relatively higher rates. Was this due to the greater participation of doctors, or, as some people have suggested because the middle-class fertility rate was lower and so they were more likely to be a primigravida and therefore more 'at risk'? Also middle-class women are more likely to become mothers at a later age and so increase the chance of birth complications and abnormalities. This pattern is true today, and the older the mother the greater the risk of giving birth to a baby with Down's Syndrome. In fact, many more babies with Down's Syndrome are born to young mothers, as more young women have babies but it is an interesting debate and the reader might consider why young women are not offered screening routinely.

The social trend in Britain for the middle classes to delay childbirth to a later stage in their lives is explained by some sociologists in *cultural* terms.

The wealthier middle class have traditionally experienced more control and autonomy in their lives. They have had more choice in many aspects of social life including education, occupation and housing. This control has extended to the deliberate planning of families. The professional middle classes were the first group to limit their families by artificial contraception in the late nineteenth century and this social class pattern of *planned* childbirth as we have seen, still remains to a lesser extent. The idea of increased control can be said to be the motivation behind the movement for the 'de-hospitalisation' of childbirth. Choice and control in childbirth as Government priorities (DOH, 1993) certainly appear to stem from middle-class values and beliefs.

But if there are cultural class differences which cause different interpretations of pregnancy and childbirth, there is also a variety of ethnic cultural divisions.

Within Asian communities for instance, it is the 'norm' for female relatives only to be present at a birth with males excluded. There are also cultural expectations regarding the showing of emotions and 'sensibility' to pain. Studies have shown that the belief that Asian and Afro-Caribbean women have different reactions to pain from those of white women, are widespread. This belief, as discussed in Chapter 3, has caused some white midwives to treat Asian women in labour in a different and potentially damaging way (Bowler, 1993).

The development and use of reproductive technologies are also influenced by social factors of class and ethnicity. Fertility treatment is not 'free' and this has led to the charge that it is only the better-off who can avail themselves of this treatment. The use of surrogate mothers, given wide publicity especially in America, has been one of a social-class division, with the wealthier woman paying a poorer one to undergo pregnancy and childbirth for her. In many ways, an analogy can be drawn here with the employment of poor women as wet-nurses to wealthy families which was common practice in the nineteenth century.

Recent controversy over the use of the technique which enables parents to choose the sex of their child has highlighted the cultural preferences which, it is feared, could result in the preponderance of male babies (Kalra, 1993).

We have seen in this chapter that pregnancy and childbirth are social and cultural as well as physiological phenomena. There is not a universal experience but one which differs for women depending upon structures of class and ethnicity. There have also been changes in the way in which society as a whole has interpreted and given meaning to the act of childbirth.

It is this social meaning which a sociological analysis seeks to understand. The seemingly 'natural' event of childbirth must be placed within the context of a stratified society. There are other seemingly 'natural' conditions which sociologists would argue have been socially constructed, for not only childbirth but motherhood itself has also been the subject of sociological examination.

Case Study 4.1   Managing labour?

Marie is 15 and pregnant. She has been admitted to the local maternity hospital for induction of labour. She has had very little antenatal care because she has managed to conceal her pregnancy from everyone around her for most of the last nine months. A week ago her mother, fearing the worst, took her see the GP. Later the same day she was seen at the hospital antenatal clinic. At that visit it was estimated by ultrasonic scan that the pregnancy was at 40 weeks gestation. Now with her pregnancy thought to be 41 weeks, she has been admitted for surgical induction of labour.

Marie was very frightened and arrived on the labour ward early one morning, accompanied by a student midwife. She was clutching a small toilet bag, a towel and *Just Seventeen*, a magazine for teenagers. She was tearful and her eye make-up had run. She had black smudges around her red eyes. She was wearing a T-shirt and jeans.

The labour ward midwife asked her if she has been to the toilet today and had she opened her bowels. She looked away, shy and embarrassed, then she nodded. The midwife advised her to take off her T-shirt and to put on a hospital gown. She warned her that if she wore a nightdress it would become soiled. Marie was confused, anxious and asked when her mother would be coming in. The midwife replied that she would telephone her later and laughed, saying it was much too early to bother anyone and anyway there was not much happening yet.

Marie began to cry. The student midwife talked with her and asked what was the matter. Marie just sobbed.

The senior houseman arrived wearing a blue theatre suit, white wellington boots with splashes of blood, a theatre hat and a mask half fastened under his chin.
He explained the procedure to Maria in these words. 'I am just going to pop the baby's waters and put a little clip on to the baby's head. Then I will put a little drip into your arm; before you know it the baby will be born, okay?' Marie did not indicate her consent or seek further clarification or information.

The hospital had an active birth policy with a strict routine of two-hourly vaginal examinations, intravenous syntocinon and continuous fetal monitoring. The houseman scrubbed up and the midwife asked Marie to 'bring your knees up, heels together, and let your legs flop apart'. Marie began to scream and sob, then she was sick. She refused to obey the instructions or let anyone examine her. Her screams become louder and louder. The senior labour-ward midwife demanded to know what was being done to control the noise. An anaesthetist was summoned and epidural planned.

Someone tried to explain to Marie what was happening, but she did not appear to understand. The midwife telephoned Marie's mother and eventually the sobbing subsided.

■ Questions and discussion points

- How many examples of power and control are there in this case study?
- Who has the power and who is exerting the control over whom? Is the doctor's power, legitimate power? If so, why?
- How might a sociologist explain the circumstances that led to this scenario? (See Chapter 1, an explanation of structures and processes as part of sociological explanation.)
- Why is Marie giving birth in hospital?
- Would the care offered to Marie have been different if a home birth had been planned?
- Suggest ways in which Maria's care could be improved.
- Analyse the role of Marie, her mother, the GP, the obstetric houseman, the hospital midwife and the student midwife in this study.
- Describe some aspects of the social meaning of childbirth as indicated in this case study.

Key points

- Birth is a social event. Feminist writers believe that birth has been dominated by a patriarchal culture.
- Birth has moved from being a private event (at home) to being a public event in a hospital.
- The changing economic structure, the role of women in the workplace, and changing expectations of birth have contributed to a new social meaning of pregnancy.
- The once-private experience of birth is now publicly shared through films, television, and books.
- The move from home birth to hospital did not just happen. It was a complex series of events and changes including concerns about safety and the availability of pain relief, but feminist writers believe that it demonstrates patriarchal control of women by men.
- The medicalisation of birth has been credited with the reduction in perinatal and maternal mortality but it produces a system of care where women's psychological and emotional needs tend to be ignored and where often the woman is described in terms of functioning or malfunctioning components.
- There has been a basic error of deduction in assuming a causal relationship between rates of hospital birth and mortality statistics.
- The loss of midwives' autonomy was associated with the growth in hospital birth and paralleled by a corresponding rise in the number and status of male obstetricians coinciding with the medicalisation of birth.
- The House of Commons Social Services Committee Report was the first

Government statement suggesting a reversal in the current trends and the need to see birth as a more natural event.

- Issues of choice and control are inextricably linked with the medicalisation of childbirth.
- Birth is a complex social and cultural experience.
- Choice and control in childbirth depend on effective communication between midwives and women. Where there is continuity of carer, communication is improved. Where communication is effective the woman is more likely to feel in control of the birth experience.

Chapter 5

Social aspects of motherhood

The focus of this chapter is an analysis of what has been called in sociology the 'myth of motherhood'. When sociologists use the word 'myth' in this context, it means that a phenomenon such as motherhood which is a reality and not fictitious in any way, is given a significance and use as a means of organising societal norms of behaviour, on a universal basis. In other words, a *social* status is endowed with a supernatural meaning and something which is historically and societally *specific* is elevated to a position of an everlasting and eternal truth. Motherhood denotes a specific biological and emotional relationship but has attained a status within society which extends beyond this basic description. Motherhood has long been culturally assumed to be the state to which all 'natural' women aspire. Motherhood, like other ideological constructs, has taken on the appearance of a 'natural' phenomenon but, as we have argued, the primary action of sociology is to be sceptical of any claim to 'natural' behaviour and to analyse social action in terms of its meaning in a specific society at a specific time and place.

Sara Delamont summarised this dominant cultural view and indicated the contradictions and absurdities which an ideology such as motherhood can contain when placed under a sociological scalpel:

> All rational, adult women want to be mothers in wedlock, so all married women want babies, and no unmarried women do. This basic belief leads to a series of correlated ideas, so that the 'problem' of the unmarried mother is 'solved' if she marries; that married women who do not want children are 'unnatural' or ill or 'selfish'; and socially most crucial, that because women are 'driven' to maternity by biological urges, all offspring of married women are 'really' wanted. (Delamont, 1980, p. 198)

These series of ideas or assumptions are held together, however illogically, with the acceptance of a 'natural' maternal instinct which is possessed by all real or 'natural' women. But this immediately begs the question, is this true of all women and if so, what of single women? If a maternal instinct is inborn why should not single women be mothers? As we shall see later, the attitude towards single motherhood has ranged historically from outright condemnation and persecution to tolerance but also resentment if they are seen to have more social advantages than 'proper' married mothers.

In the previous chapter, we looked at pregnancy and childbirth as social and cultural conditions as well as biological ones. Likewise motherhood and, to a lesser extent, fatherhood, are both essentially socially defined, limited and constructed patterns of behaviour which have the appearance of some form of 'natural' instinct.

In this chapter we are concerned to look at five main strands in the social meaning of 'motherhood':

1. the sociological and historical construction of motherhood within which the position of single motherhood is historically examined, the question of the individual's 'right' to motherhood and the power which it confers, and the way in which the state has defined this role;
2. motherhood as a fulfilling and socially enhancing experience Is this true for all women? We analyse the debate on the causes of post-natal depression;
3. the creation of 'good' and 'bad' mothers and the concept of bonding;
4. motherhood and sexuality. Is motherhood an essentially sexless state or the ultimate signification of femininity and what is the cultural relationship between sexuality and motherhood?
5. fatherhood. What is the role for fathers in the late twentieth century? What is a 'good' father?

■ Motherhood as a social and historical construct

If women are believed to have a basic and inborn maternal instinct, this is in complete contrast to men who are not assumed to have a natural paternal instinct. On the other hand, men are at the mercy of uncontrollable and easily aroused sexual drives which 'cause' them to behave in ways which although regrettable, are not really their fault. This seemingly all-powerful masculine sex drive has often been cited as the justification for rape, and the necessity for prostitution as a social service which protects 'good' women. So the connected statuses of motherhood and fatherhood are not only defined differently in our society, they carry very different rights, assumptions and expected behaviour patterns and are treated differently in law and social policies. In Chapter 7 we will see how the policies of the British state have, over time, constructed and defined the roles of mother and father and constructed a model of 'the family' upon which British welfare policy is based.

The first step in an analysis of such a culturally dominant idea as motherhood is to ask how such an idea is transmitted in a society. Images of motherhood are to be found throughout art, popular culture, literature and religion. The phrase itself evokes much more than just a biological description, when we talk of 'mothering' it implies a relationship based upon caring, responsibility and to a certain extent, self-sacrifice. On the other hand, to 'father' a child, carries a totally different connotation: one based almost solely on a physical act of procreation and potential authority. It is through looking at the meaning we place upon everyday words in our language that we begin to gain an insight into their *social meaning*. These social meanings are evident in the use of the words 'mother' and 'father' in everyday language. We talk of someone as a 'mother-figure' and this implies a person who gives security and warmth, but a 'father-figure' is one of kindly authority who offers protection.

We can see therefore that the roles of mother and father are endowed with different sets of expectations and beliefs but it is important to remember that there is nothing 'natural' about these assumptions, they are specific to a historical time, place and culture.

Anthropologists such as Margaret Mead (1950) have chronicled the ways in which different societies have defined the roles of mother and father. Some societies negate the role of father altogether with the mother's brother taking on the responsibility for bringing up his nephews and nieces. The Matebele of Zimbabwe do not have a word in their language for a biological mother, for she and all her sisters are viewed as mothers of the same child. As we shall see in the following section, within British society both in the past and present, definitions of 'motherhood' differ between social classes and ethnic groups. The task of sociology is to hold up seemingly obvious concepts such as motherhood to a bright light of scrutiny and in British society this has been undertaken largely by feminist scholarship in the recent past. 'Motherhood' is not a concept with an unequivocal and given meaning: it has been given a specific meaning and definition by society. This meaning is, however, always shot through with contradictions and has to be constantly reinforced and redefined. One of the basic contradictions within our society is that the status of motherhood is hedged around by qualifications.

☐ **Motherhood and marriage**

The dominant view in British society remains that married motherhood is vastly preferable to unmarried motherhood for ideological, social and economic reasons. Until fairly recently the status of an unmarried mother was one which most girls even of the generation growing up in the 1950s and 1960s viewed with dread and horror. There was only one remedy for this terrible state – marriage. As Table 5.1 demonstrates, the incidence of births to teenage women was higher during the 1960s than at present, but the great difference over the past thirty years has been the rejection of marriage as an outcome of pregnancy.

This rise in unmarried motherhood as a choice is one which is unique in the social history of the past two centuries. As Britain became an

Table 5.1 Non-marital births, adoptions and abortions, England and Wales, 1959–84

Year	Non-marital births	Children adopted by non-parents	Ratio of non-parent adoptions to non-marital births	Legal abortions (1000)*
1959	38 161	7 966	20.9	–
1960	42 707	9 064	21.2	–
1961	48 490	10 065	10.8	–
1962	55 376	11 046	19.9	–
1963	59 104	11 644	19.7	–
1964	63 340	13 470	21.3	–
1965	66 249	13 631	20.6	–
1966	67 065	14 106	21.0	–
1967	69 928	14 222	20.3	–
1968	69 806	14 751	21.1	21.2
1969	67 041	13 129	19.6	26.9
1970	64 744	10 797	16.7	41.7
1971	65 678	9 642	14.7	53.0
1972	62 511	8 170	13.1	61.7
1973	58 100	7 388	12.7	63.8
1974	56 500	6 621	11.7	64.2
1975	54 900	5 774	10.5	63.1
1976	53 800	4 777	8.9	61.6
1977	55 400	4 026	7.3	63.0
1978	60 700	3 926	6.3	69.0
1979	69 500	3 539	5.1	77.3
1980	77 400	3 529	4.6	84.7
1981	81 000	3 270	4.0	86.2
1982	89 900	3 284	3.7	87.8
1983	99 200	3 008	3.0	87.2
1984	110 500	2 910	2.6	96.1

* Single, widowed, divorced and separated women only.

Sources: Statistical Review of England and Wales for the years 1958 to 1973; OPCS Monitor 1976–1984; Abortion Statistics (Series AB), 1974–84; Selmen (1994). Reproduced by permission.

industrial society with a growing urban population so institutions were developed to control the poor and the criminal classes – the 'dangerous classes' as they were named. Unmarried mothers were defined as female delinquents of questionable mental ability and the very state of unmarried motherhood was associated with ideas of moral degeneracy. This resulted in the incarceration of women in workhouses and asylums for no other reason than that they were 'unsupported' and pregnant. Crowther (1981) has shown that women made up the bulk of inmates in workhouses after the Poor Law of 1834, and that the majority of these women were aged between 16 and 40, male inmates were more likely to be over 40 with the majority being over 60. This gives us a new insight into the functions of workhouses – they were basically institutions for unmarried mothers. Towards the end of the nineteenth century homes specialising in 'rescue' work with unmarried mothers and their children were founded and many of these were still in existence in the 1960s. The purpose of these homes was twofold; to redeem the sinful mother and to make sure that she 'earned her forgiveness' and to provide a source of adoption for the children. When a mother was incarcerated in a workhouse her child was frequently separated from her and given for fostering 'to learn a trade' or for adoption.

Because illegitimacy was regarded as a sign of 'feeble-mindedness' the concern for the child was not widely felt and the survival of the child 'born in sin' was seen as of little importance to respectable society. The mortality rate for illegitimate children was always much higher than for legitimate ones and the death rate of children who were sent to 'baby farms' can only be guessed at. But in the two years between 1860 and 1862 there were officially recorded 902 'infant murders' in England and Wales (Smith, 1979).

One of the occupations open to unmarried mothers which would save them from destitution and the workhouse, was that of wet-nurse. This was a job which paid relatively well, involved the woman being lodged in the house of the rich family employing her and of course she was assured of a good diet whilst breast-feeding. This also meant that her own recently born child must have been 'accommodated' elsewhere. The history of infanticide and 'neglect' in Victorian society is a deeply shocking one (Smith, 1979) and it was illegitimate children, because of the enforced poverty and social ostracisation of the mother, who formed the majority of the victims. The practice of wet-nursing is an interesting one when placed within the ideology of motherhood. It was also widely believed that characteristics such as goodness and kindness were 'imbibed with the mother's milk' and yet numbers of the wealthy turned their babies over to labelled 'degenerates' for nursing!

The stigma of illegitimacy and single motherhood slowly declined throughout the twentieth century but the National Birthrate Commission which was set up after the 1914–18 war recommended that the Endowment for Motherhood (the forerunner of the Family Allowance) which they were demanding, should only be paid to married mothers.

Although much of the stigma of being an unmarried mother has to a certain extent lessened in the past twenty years they are still seen as a 'social problem'. As recently as 1995 there have been demands from a group of right-wing Conservatives for a return to hostels for unmarried mothers and for their babies to be placed for adoption. But why does the prospect of unmarried motherhood seem to pose such a danger to the social order?

A feminist perspective would argue that it is seen as a threat by a patriarchal culture which defines women as passive and dependent beings and therefore the sign of an independent motherhood which exists without a male figure undermines all authority structures. However, the problem of the connection between poverty and unmarried motherhood is one which still remains today.

On the other hand, 'working' mothers constitute another category of a social problem and debates rage over the desirability of mother-care versus other forms of child-care. But despite these caveats, 'motherhood' does carry a certain cultural status for women within the state welfare and legislative system.

As we shall see in Chapter 7, it is as mothers that women enter into certain citizenship rights such as the receipt of child benefit, preference in housing applications and, possibly, more lenient prison sentencing. But on the other hand, they face discrimination in employment and education, more surveillance by health and welfare agencies and limitations on participation in training and pension schemes and are penalised by the tax system.

☐ Learning to be a mother

To argue that motherhood is a social construct means that it must be seen as *learned behaviour* within a society's norms and structures. How do young women learn what motherhood means, and how have successive generations been socialised into the concept of successful mothering?

One way in which this information has been transmitted has been to convert motherhood from a 'natural' instinct (not to be confused with maternal desire to give birth physically) to a skill which has to be taught. Childbearing may remain a basic physical and biological phenomenon but child-rearing has been expanded into a science which requires professional expertise. As Diane Richardson (1993) has recently chronicled, advice on how to bring up children had become big business in Western countries by the middle of this century. Advice on the 'correct' methods of feeding, disciplining, and schedules for rest and play have changed between the 1920s and the present day, so that the 'correct' method of, say, feeding at strict times was superseded in the 1960s by advice to 'feed on demand', so what constituted 'good' mothering for one generation was overturned for the next. One interesting fact that emerges from Diane Richardson's study is the fact that until about thirty years ago almost all the books on child-rearing were written by men! It is only comparatively recently that writers such as Miriam Stoppard (1984) and Penelope Leach (1984) have become child-rearing gurus.

Many of the theories on child-rearing have their basis in psychology, and the theories of Freud and specifically of the influential 'maternal deprivation' argument of John Bowlby (1953) which gained great credence during the 1950s and 1960s have been criticised by feminist writers as a patriarchal ideology which serves to limit and control women's activities. Radical feminist psychologists such as Nancy Chodorow have, in recent years, attempted to rework theories on maternal child-rearing into a feminist perspective (Chodorow, 1994). We will discuss some of these in more depth later in this chapter. What this proliferation of child-rearing manuals and psychological theories have shown however, is that mothering cannot be taken for granted as a natural instinct, it has to be carefully taught.

But as we stressed earlier, a sociological analysis must take into account the variations within a society between different social groups, so before looking in more depth at some of the theories of maternal bonding, we will look at some of these cultural and socio-economic differences in aspects of motherhood.

☐ **The 'right' to be a mother**

Do all women have the 'right' to be a mother? In the past, childlessness was a state which many women may have regretted but felt was beyond their power to alter. But with the development of reproductive technologies, motherhood is increasingly seen as a real individual 'choice'. Childlessness may now be defined as being within a woman's power to determine. As a recent survey reported (HMSO, 1995) more and more women are actively choosing not to be mothers. If this trend continues, it is estimated that one in eight women born in the 1980s will choose to be childless. The birth rate is falling, and at present levels will not replace the UK population.

Therefore increasingly childlessness is seen as something which is chosen rather than imposed. What does this mean for those who wish to remain childless? Ideologically they are still often defined as 'selfish' or 'unnatural'. The advent and limited availability of fertility treatment has changed the *social meaning* of the childless woman. She can now be seen not as someone to be pitied but as someone who has either chosen this state (selfish) or has not been 'successful' in receiving treatment.

The technical possibility of 'curing' infertility has, it has been argued, reinforced the ideology of the 'natural' maternal instinct. As Michelle Stanworth has argued, it makes women who do not seek treatment appear to be peculiar or disturbed. She quotes Patrick Steptoe, the obstetrician who pioneered the first 'test tube baby', as saying, 'It is a fact that there is a biological drive to reproduce. Women who deny this drive, or in whom it is frustrated show disturbances in other ways' (Stanworth, 1987, p. 15). In addition to the reinforcement of the ideology of motherhood, fertility treatment has also been criticised by sociologists and feminists for its cultural emphasis on 'success' and also consumerism. IVF treatment is often held up as the way in which couples can become a 'success'. As Taylor (1990) quotes an American obstetrician as saying, 'Our culture worships success and denigrates the quitter'(1990, p. 773). This emphasis on the success in gaining a baby is further reinforced by some of the language used in advertising the delights of parenthood.

This is an example of a particularly emotive advertisement from a private clinic, 'There is no other perfume like it, the smell of the newborn: a milk scent, warm scent cuddle essence' (Foster, 1995, p. 57). Not only is this a wildly inaccurate picture, it is also playing on the vulnerability of women who are childless.

A sociological perspective would ask, why has infertility become a 'problem'? Is it because the problem itself has been constructed by the very technology which has been developed? In other words, infertility which has always existed in a minority of women, has suddenly been defined as 'problematic' because there exists a scientific and technological remedy. What did women do about infertility before the technological 'fix' was available?

The 'desperation' of infertile couples has been the way in which the press and popular media have carried the message of the success of treatment. Sarah Franklin (1990), has deconstructed this use of 'desperation' in the popular discourse surrounding fertility treatment. Note that it is always 'couples' who are 'desperate', never single or lesbian women! The success of the treatment is always given wide publicity although, of course, the actual success rate is very small. The majority of infertile couples who undergo techniques such as IVF and GIFT still fail to produce a healthy child. By the end of the 1980s the overall success rate in well-established IVF clinics was only 9.7 per cent per couple treated (Foster, 1995).

How then can we 'understand' the development of fertility treatment? Is it a means by which the obstetric profession can regain some measure of power and control over a new 'patient population' within a society with a falling birth rate? Is it an illustration of a reactionary ideology surrounding the 'naturalness' of motherhood?

In a sense, the availability of IVF treatment illustrates the social class and ethnic divisions within society. Because of its limited availability within the Health Service, much of the treatment is only a 'choice' for wealthier couples. It is also axiomatic that the woman is within a marriage or a steady relationship and preferably of white 'respectable' social status. One woman was refused IVF treatment because she had a previous conviction for prostitution; this was challenged in the courts but the medical decision to withhold treatment was upheld. The RCOG in 1983 stated that treatment can be refused on social as well as medical grounds, and that single women should not be treated (RCOG, 1983).

We can see therefore that the development of technologies do not eradicate existing ideas about the gender roles which are deemed 'natural' but, in fact, can be used to reinforce them. The state of childlessness in a (married) woman is still viewed as a problem to be cured or as a sign of mental disturbance. Nowhere is this more clear than in the widely held belief that in cases of baby abduction the culprit is likely to be a woman who has recently 'lost' a child or who cannot have a baby. Police investigations are predicated upon this psychological portrait and yet recent research (Channel 4, 1995), has shown that this is far from the truth. Most women who abduct a child are in an unsatisfactory relationship and see a child as a means of improving this but their partners are unwilling or judged as 'unready' to undertake parenthood.

Motherhood is desired by probably the vast majority of women. Does it therefore confer a measure of social status and power?

☐ **Class, ethnicity and matriarchal power**

Motherhood and the individual meaning given to being a mother is not a uniform and universal social experience. However, there are differences between social-class and ethnic groups. So as well as changing historically within British society and the dominant culture as a whole, there also exist fragmented and opposing definitions of motherhood, its requirements and the power which it confers.

Traditionally there existed extensive class differences in the role which mothers were expected to play. For upper-class and aristocratic families the role of mother in the sense of actual 'hands-on' caring and 'mothering' was practically non-existent. Wives were expected to produce an heir but not actually to look after their children. These tasks were allocated to an army of female domestic servants including the all-important figure of 'nanny'. Aristocratic children were 'nannied' rather than 'mothered'. It was the professional, qualified and experienced nanny (of a lower class) who was responsible for child-rearing, not the biological mother. The successful aristocratic mother was one who had first produced at least two male heirs, 'one heir and one to spare', followed possibly by a daughter or two and who was efficient in being primarily a good hostess and an efficient household manager. Sons were sent off to school at as early an age as 8, and so were seen only for a short time every year and daughters were assigned to the jurisdiction of maids, nannies and governesses until such time as they 'came out' in society to be married to a suitable man and then move out to begin their own household. It is interesting to note that the same maternal distance and separation from children among the lower classes was termed as 'neglect' and children were said to be suffering from maternal deprivation.

Did motherhood confer a power status upon aristocratic women? The answer to this question is hedged with qualifications, certainly to be the mother of male heirs was all-important – after all if she continually produced daughters, she could be regarded as a failure. In some circumstances this was the cause of divorce (the cases of Henry VIII and, more recently, of the ex-Shah of Persia spring to mind) and this remains the case in other cultures until the present. But the power of aristocratic women and indeed of queens did not rest upon their status of mother but upon other factors of inheritance, independent wealth and marriage.

Within most working-class cultures the view of the mother as the all-powerful matriarch within the home was pervasive but also needs perhaps a closer scrutiny. As Wilmott and Young (1960) chronicled in their study of the extended family network in London in the 1950s, the primary relationship of this structure was that of mother and daughter. Children were more often seen as a wider familial responsibility with grandmother and aunts taking on some of the child-care role from the individual mother. This support network of the extended family has in recent years been regarded as a more liberating influence than the individualistic child-centred nuclear family structure (Greer, 1985). It must also be remembered that in the absence of universal nursery and crèche provision, the bulk of child care for working mothers is undertaken by grandmothers and other relatives. But children are seen as primarily the responsibility of the biological mother in all aspects of everyday life. Health visitors focus upon her, as do school communications; most GPs expect the mother to bring children to the surgery; it is mothers who are expected to stay in hospital with sick children. But does this responsibility confer power upon her?

Autobiographies of male working-class writers like Richard Hoggart (1955) and Robert Roberts (1973) paint perhaps a rather masculine and romanticised view of the poor and self-sacrificing mother who was the pivot of the home. But what is the basis for a matriarchal power? A Marxist argument would stress that all power must stem from an economic base, whereas a Weberian view would be that of power in class and status groups. Foucault would see the diversity of power as being reinforced constantly through subjective personal relationships. In some ways, all these analyses can be applied to an understanding and calculation of matriarchal power. Wilmott and Young (although not Marxists) placed the basis for the matriarchal power of the East End mother to her control over housing in the form of her named tenancy of the house, her relative economic independence, and on her authority over daughters and children. But in many regional cultures the sphere of the power of the mother only extends to the front-door; women may have power over household decisions concerning children but not over decisions affecting the outside world. It is 'private' rather than 'public' power.

Does the status of 'mother' itself confer any purchase on power, and how much power should a mother possess? Mothers must not be seen to exercise too much power, after all the 'dominant mother' is often blamed for the incidence of schizophrenia or even homosexuality in sons.

Over whom is this power exercised? Mothers may have a degree of power over their own children but this is by its very nature of a short-term duration, but a mother will not have power over other people's children.

Even within a two-parent home, a mother's power will frequently be seen as of a subordinate nature to that of the father. 'Wait till your father gets home!' was the ultimate appeal to a higher authority. The amount of economic power a mother may hold is not therefore dependent upon motherhood but upon many other social and economic reasons. It could be said that motherhood confers a high *ideological* status but a correspondingly low *economic* status. We will return to this point later when looking at some of the social reasons for post-natal depression.

Within ethnic cultures, motherhood is given varying definitions. Commentators have frequently claimed that 'black' and Asian families , have for differing reasons, been designated as 'pathological' by social welfare agencies (Guru, 1986; Owusu-Bempah, 1989; Gilroy, 1987). Within many Asian cultures motherhood does confer a status to a woman who is the mother of sons but usually this power position is only gained at an older age over daughters-in-law and is, of course, dependent upon the production of sons as daughters are 'lost' to the family of the husband (Werbner, 1989; Bhachu, 1985). This is, in contrast to a widely held view within an English culture (and often reflected in social policies and care organisation) that it is daughters who remain close to home and who will provide care in old age whilst sons are expected to move away.

Among the traditional Jewish culture, mothers exert a wide degree of power and authority which is extended to the primacy of the mother as the determinant of Jewish religious and cultural belonging. Jewishness is traced through the maternal and not the paternal line of descent.

As we can see, the status conferred by motherhood is a very complex tangle to unravel, but the identification of the rights and responsibilities of motherhood have been systematically set out in social policies and legislation.

☐ The state and motherhood

Historically, motherhood has not always been endowed with the importance that it has achieved in this century. Donzelot (1980) in his Foucauldian account of the growth in the intervention by the state into the realm of family life argued that it was during the period of industrial capitalist development in the nineteenth century that the role of motherhood became defined and set by state legislation. It was during this period that agents of the state from health, social welfare and education began to set out what was required from women as mothers. This had a twin effect of subjecting them to surveillance by the state via health visitors, doctors and teachers but at the same time it also elevated the status of mother within the family. Thus it was, argues Donzelot, that mothers became the organising agents of state policy within society and the State came to replace the power of the father over family life and installed the mother as the chief agent of control over families.

In Britain, by the latter decades of the nineteenth century there was a move by the state to become more interventionist and to take an active role in the health and welfare of children. Writers such as Anna Davin (1978) and Jane Lewis (1980) have argued that this stance was adopted against the background of the high rate of infant mortality and fear of the 'decline of the British race'. These concerns were fuelled by the need to supply 'soldiers for the Empire' and the economic requirements for a large labour force. Policies on education and the introduction of compulsory and free schooling ran parallel to the measures on health and welfare. The person of the working-class mother became the object of state policies and the attention of health and social workers. She was, at the same time, the person held to blame for the high rate of infant mortality through her ignorance and fecklessness and she was also to be the agent of change.

Health visiting, which was a new occupation for women, targeted working-class women as the objects of attention. Schools for Mothers were set up in many areas and Maternal and Child Welfare clinics were set up by local authorities under state legislation in 1919. This attitude by the health and social welfare organisations persists to the present time with nearly all the healthy eating and health education messages aimed specifically at mothers who are officially seen as the persons with the main responsibility for children.

This 'official' definition has become a *normative* ideology, so that when a mother does not perform this caring role she is perceived as deviant or abnormal. Even when the ambiguous word 'parent' is used in notices the informal and intended meaning is that it is the mother who is really being addressed. It is mothers who are naturally expected to stay with children in hospital; most health visitors and GPs still expect the mother to bring a child for injections or for check-ups; it is not unknown for some schools still to expect mothers to be at home or at least 'to be available' via a contact number during the day if an emergency should occur during school hours.

Ideologies on a 'woman's place' and the natural instinct for motherhood have been reflected in state policies. It was as a mother that women attained a measure of citizenship status within the growth of state intervention this century. In the Beveridge Report of 1942 it was as wives and mothers that women entered into the social welfare system, with their entitlement to a restricted range of benefits dependent upon this position and gained through the payments made by the male partner. Interestingly, the only state benefit to which women are entitled as of right is the child benefit which is dependent upon the status of mother. We will return in Chapter 7, to a discussion on the way in which single mothers have become on one hand the targets of condemnation and on the other are seen as having preferential treatment in the social welfare system.

We began this chapter by stating that 'motherhood' has been identified by some sociologists as an ideological concept. This interpretation has emerged from a broadly feminist school of sociological scholarship (Gittins, 1985). Within an older tradition of sociology, the definition and meaning of motherhood went largely unchallenged within the framework of studies of the sociology of 'the family'. By the 1970s critiques of the 'norm' of the nuclear family emerged from radical psychiatry (Laing, 1971; Cooper, 1972) which attacked the structure of the family as potentially destructive to individuals. This critique was paralleled within sociology by the 'sociology of knowledge' school which focused upon an analysis of the production of knowledge within society (Lovell, 1980; Berger and Berger, 1983). This type of analysis located forms of knowledge within the social power structures of society and argued against the 'objective' and free-floating definition of knowledge. Assumptions about the 'naturalness' of institutions and structures were being widely questioned.

Feminism took 'the family' as an institution to be analysed and questioned in terms of its impact on the lives of women (Barrett and McIntosh, 1982; Delphy, 1977). These analyses questioned above all the 'natural' status of gendered divisions of labour within the home and the division between private and public spheres (Harris, 1981). Much of this work revolved around a growing interest in ideology stemming from debates in sociology on the work of Louis Althusser (1970) concerning the role of 'Ideological State Apparatuses' (ISAs) of which the family was one. This work formed the theoretical framework for a feminist analysis of women and welfare (Wilson, 1977) and had an influence on the whole field of study on a 'familial ideology' (Beechey, 1985).

The definition of 'motherhood' within the familial ideology took on the appearance of naturalness. This is the real strength of an ideology. Its dominance means that for many women the pressure to conform to the tightly restricted definition of motherhood is almost overpowering. One result is that some women may feel guilt if they cannot 'measure up' to the standards which they believe are 'natural' and unquestionable. This classification of a definition of motherhood as being socially constructed and not based upon 'objective' knowledge lies at the heart of a sociological explanation of post-natal depression.

■ A social understanding of post-natal depression

We referred earlier in the chapter to the contradiction between the relatively high ideological status given to motherhood and the correspondingly low economic status which it confers. This argument is often employed when looking at some of the social factors involved in the incidence of post-natal depression. Having a baby is a form of economic suicide. It almost inevitably leads to a halving of income and a doubling of expenditure. It is not an activity to be taken on lightly by those who value their freedom and financial security associated with that freedom. Kitzinger (1980) describes the adjustment in these terms:

> Psychologically, the first months after birth are a time in which great adjustments are necessary. The mother – even though she hesitates to admit it often harbours a secret resentment against the baby who has deprived her of her freedom and the leisure of bachelor girl life . . .
> Now she may have no money of her own, no personal allowance and no joint bank account, she has to squeeze money for her clothes, her personal luxuries and presents from housekeeping money. She feels tied down by maternity and domesticity. She struggles with tasks for which she has not been trained and which recur day after day with monotonous regularity. She longs to be the carefree girl she once was and this desire makes her feel guilty and adds further to the strain.
> (Kitzinger, 1980)

Most midwifery texts define three types of emotional or mental disturbances following childbirth as, post natal blues, post-natal depression and puerperal psychosis (Silverton, 1993; Cox, 1986). Post-natal depression is said to affect up to 10 per cent of women following childbirth. Pitt (1968) describes post-natal depression as being accompanied by tearfulness, despondency, feelings of inadequacy, inability to cope, feelings of anxiety about the baby and guilt linked to self-reproach at care perceived as inadequate. There have been many studies (Pitt, 1968; Dalton, 1980) that have demonstrated that post-natal depression is unlike depression at other stages of women's lives and more recently Cox *et al.* (1993) have concluded that post-natal illness 'is a direct consequence of the physical and psychological stresses of childbirth'. Ball (1994) in her excellent book, *Reactions to Motherhood*, describes some of the early studies of emotional outcomes of childbirth. She says:

> It is intriguing to note that certain early studies of 'maladjustment' to motherhood sought to explain women's reactions in terms of their 'femininity'. In a description of maternal emotions, Newton (1955) explored the feelings of women towards menstruation, pregnancy and childbirth, breast-feeding, caring for an infant and 'other aspects of femininity' with a clear inference that 'feminine' women would feel positive about these experiences. (Ball, 1994, p. 18)

She quotes Chertok (1969) and Nilsson (1972) who both produced scales of 'femininity' from which they attempted to show that post-natal depression was related to a woman's rejection of her feminine role in childbirth.

Kitzinger (1992) argues that in Western cultures when a woman is distressed after having a baby, who feels cheated, or feels she has failed a vital test of womanhood is likely to be told she is suffering from post-natal depression. The problem is caused by a malfunctioning component, in this case a faulty endocrine gland or a personality defect. She argues that in a technological culture such as this, it is doctors who define birth and women who experience it. She believes that traditional explanations of unhappiness are based on the medical model of birth that places the blame on the woman and her 'faulty functioning'. Kitzinger (1992), like Ball (1994), believes that there are many causes of unhappiness in woman's lives including socio-economic problems, poverty, unemployment, poor living conditions, domestic violence, and lack of support. Kitzinger (1990) also describes how a crying baby can quickly shatter emotional stability when there is no extended family around to offer respite and support. She also recounts how some women describe their experience of birth as rape and with such descriptions it is not difficult to understand post-natal depression nor to put it in a more appropriate context. Clement (1995) examined the research evidence to ascertain whether 'listening visits' in pregnancy, targeted at women with low emotional well-being would be effective in preventing post-natal depression and improving other psychological outcomes. She concluded that many women depressed after childbirth were also depressed in pregnancy and that someone to talk to and someone to listen to may benefit many women who experience depression alongside childbirth. This in an interesting paper that does not assume that post-natal depression has a simple physical cause. The intervention of a midwife as a compassionate, informed, knowledgable and supportive friend, it seems, can help women.

The birth of a baby is a time of great stress, change and is associated with the loss of the old order of things. It is clear that some women are simply mourning the loss of a previous life style. There is much in the literature on grief and loss which helps in understanding post-natal depressive illness as a social construct. Worden (1991) describes the four tasks of mourning as:

- *To accept the reality of the loss.* This can be translated in motherhood to accepting the reality of pregnancy and the realisation that life will never be the same again.
- *To work through the pain of grief.* In childbirth this may be the physical, emotional and psychological pain of childbirth as well as the pain associated with the loss of a previous life-style, status or position.
- *To adjust to the environment where the deceased is missing.* This is adjusting to a new environment where a dependent individual makes new and sometimes excessive demands on the physically and emotional exhausted mother.
- *To emotionally relocate the deceased and move on with life.* Women are

required to move on with life immediately. There is no time to mourn the life that has past, only the work of the new.

Even the long 'lying in period' where women had a chance to rest has been usurped by the need to go shopping or clean the house. Moving on often happens more rapidly than many women want and depression may be a chance to slow the pace. This is another explanation for post-natal depression. To assume that post-natal illness is simply a physical disease of the body with a faulty component is to ignore the social aspects of motherhood.

■ 'Good' and 'bad' mothers and bonding

What makes a woman a 'good' or a 'bad' mother? Many psychological theories of maternal bonding and the importance of the mother in child development have been criticised by feminist writers as having a restrictive and controlling effect on women's perceptions and behaviour.

Feminist critics such as Williams and Watson (1988) have argued that many of these ideas have become a part of accepted knowledge within social work and that the growth of family therapy techniques and practices have served to further 'victimise' mothers in so-called 'problem' families. 'Bad' mothers can be punished by the state, by having their children taken away from them. Not only are many of these theories taken on board without any recognition of class or ethnic and cultural differences, they are also based upon the assumption that the traditional family forms and gender roles are inherently superior and therefore should be the model to which all should aspire.

A view which goes directly against the 'good' mothering argument is that of Nancy Chodorow (1994) a radical feminist psychologist who argued that the fact that it is women who have been allocated the mothering tasks in most modern societies is crucial to our understanding of the differences in orientation between males and females and is to the detriment of both. She puts forward the view that boys learn what it is to be masculine by comparing their parents and then distancing themselves from what they know is 'feminine' – their mother. The development of masculinity therefore, is predicated upon that which is not female, so any so-called feminine characteristics are severely rejected by boys in their definition of masculine behaviour. On the other hand, girls learn what is 'feminine' by comparing themselves and conforming to the figure of their mother. Boys learn to distance themselves and girls to compare and conform to the expectations of others like themselves. This pattern would be negated, argues Chodorow, if mothering became a more shared activity between men and women. According to Nicolson (1993) the notion of maternal instinct underpins the contemporary construct of motherhood.

She argues that it underlines notions of femininity and what is perceived as 'required maternal behaviour'. Nicolson believes an absence of this so-called maternal instinct is used to explain women's 'failures' as mothers when their children are neglected in some way.

Bonding is yet another myth of motherhood. Good mothers bond well and develop their 'maternal instinct', then they become the best mothers. 'Bad' mothering can thus be explained by the woman's failure to bond with her child and the lack of maternal instinct. Whatever the outcome mothers are 'blamed' and seen as powerful and destructive simultaneously (Nicolson, 1993).

Bonding or parental-infant attachment theories have emerged from the work of Bowlby (1953) and others who argued that this crucial relationship between mother (not the father or siblings) and child is established around the time of birth. Bowlby believed that if this bonding process was disrupted in any way, by separation, or insensitive maternity care, then the mother would fail to bond with the baby and subsequently fail to nurture the child appropriately. Klaus and Kennell (1976) described an acutely sensitive period at or soon after birth when mother–baby bonding should occur. Bowlby's theories have been criticised by a number of authors including MacFarlane (1984) and Eyer (1993) who believe that although it is important for a good relationship to be established between the child and the parent it is not necessary for this to occur at the time of birth. Bowlby (1953) also believed that mothers' love was essential to health and these studies led to theories of maternal deprivation. Women were to care for children, provide a firm stable base, and be available at all times. These theories influenced child-care and state social policy in Britain.

Good mothers are thus defined as those mothers who have established a good relationship with their child at birth and continue to provide this intimate care as and when it is needed. This enables them always to put their child first and conform to the acceptable standards of motherhood. Bad or 'problem' mothers, are held responsible for most, if not all, morbidity in their children. According to Liptak *et al.* (1983) 'Interventions which increase the competence of parents and improve their sensitivity to their children, can be expected to decrease the occurrence of these problems.' Thus it would seem that bad mothers (not parents) who coincidentally have often failed 'to bond' with their child, and by definition have a poorly developed 'maternal instinct' are those who are incompetent, go out to work, employ child-minders, have children who have problems with behaviour and are emotionally deprived. Their children are abused or neglected, they live in poor-quality housing on large estates, and also act in ways that demonstrate that they have failed to establish a caring relationship. They also have children on 'at risk' registers and are likely to be unsupported. Popular rhetoric would have us believe that they are subsequently more likely to injure and abuse their children (Lynch and Roberts, 1977), fail to protect them from accidents and allow them to suffer from infectious diseases. Motherhood is an awesome responsibility!

Bonding as a theory has been accepted generally without question by those wishing to improve the care in maternity hospitals. In the past strict regimes separated mothers and babies for hours and even days after birth and for ill-defined reasons. The bonding theory was used in presenting the case for humanising many maternity units and for this it has been beneficial.

In summary and according to Nicolson (1993) the role of 'mother' has not just evolved in a natural way, outside culture and free from ideology. It has been socially constructed within patriarchy through a complex set of power relations which ensure that women become mothers, and practice motherhood in narrowly defined ways.

■ Motherhood and sexuality

The state of motherhood is obviously bound up with definitions of sexuality. The interlinking of sexual identity, sexual activity and mother-hood is a very complex tangle to unpick. The reason why the state of pregnancy was the subject of shame and secrecy in the past, was that it proclaimed evidence of sexual activity which, for women, was regarded very ambivalently. It meant that even 'nice' women who were safely and respectably married had engaged in sexual intercourse.

But once pregnant, women also became 'sexless', once the pregnancy became obvious, most women internalised the cultural message that they had ceased to be sexually attractive or desirable. This sexless identity tended also to carry on into motherhood, it was always felt that for a mother to be sexually active was against the dominant definition of motherhood as an almost pure and unsullied state. The feminist philosopher, Marina Warner (1976), has argued that this is the basis for the Judaeo-Christian construction of the Virgin birth, that the image of the virgin mother was the epitome of masculine idealisation.

Even with all these cultural contradictions surrounding motherhood and sexuality the one basic fact remained, that all mothers are obviously heterosexual. But this is, of course simply untrue. The cases of lesbian mothers seeking custody of their children and of lesbian women seeking to adopt have, in the 1990s, become the subject of much media attention and of a legal judgement (Brophy, 1989).

According to Jackson (1993) a lesbian couple however long established have no legally recognised relationship with each other. She points out that a lesbian mother can lose custody of her children (because as a lesbian she can be defined as a bad mother) and her partner has no legally sanctioned relationship to the children. It is easy for midwives to fall into the trap of assuming that all women are heterosexual, married and happy to be mothers. Nicolson (1993) a feminist writer, argues that each of these conditions – heterosexuality, marriage and motherhood – entails a form of oppression and control, and that social class, 'race', ethnicity, sexuality and economic status further impinge upon the social conditions of mothering for individual women. This has been demonstrated in this chapter. She argues that contemporary motherhood exists within the Western patriarchal parcel of rules that control women. Thus it would seem that motherhood is not universally desirable and cannot be presumed to exist only in heterosexual marriages.

The tennis star Martina Navratilova, a self-proclaimed and much-publicised lesbian woman, recently (1994) announced her intention of having a baby on her retirement from professional sport. These examples highlight the complexity of society's definitions of both motherhood and sexuality. If motherhood is the desire of all 'natural' and 'real' women, how does one explain the lesbian mother? Either lesbianism is a part of being a 'natural' woman or motherhood is not, this is the inescapable and logical dilemma posed by a rigid definition of femininity and motherhood.

■ The social meaning of fatherhood

In Western societies, fatherhood has not attained the central ideological position which has accrued to motherhood. Men are not socialised from childhood into a role as a father. There are no comparable toys such as dolls or prams which give small boys a future model of fatherhood. Even in adult life, men are rarely given the sole identity of 'husband and father' as women are identified as 'wife and mother'. Again the language which we use is crucial in placing society's expectations of behaviour; men are described as 'a family man' because they are not 'naturally' placed in this role, women are not described as a 'family woman'. But women are described as a 'career woman' whereas men are assumed to be 'career'-orientated and so there is not an equivalent description. What then is the social meaning of fatherhood?

Sociologically, fatherhood is bound up with authority patterns, the description a *patriarchal* authority aptly defines the power which accrues to the role. Paternalism is the description given to a certain form of management or organisational structure which concentrates on the exercise of benevolent power which at the same time denies any alternative power structures. For instance, organisations which have this type of management organisation usually put into place welfare and social benefits for their staff but at the same time deny the right to belong to a trade union and install strict rules on employee behaviour. Interestingly, when her husband dies, a woman is described as a widow but her children as 'orphans' which suggests that they have no living parent.

In sociology and psychology, studies of fatherhood are rare. In sociology they tend to centre on the power dimensions within the family and gender roles. Recently, the subject of the necessity of paternal authority has surfaced in discussions on the breakdown of family life, the increase in single mothers and the connection with juvenile crime (Dennis and Erdos, 1992) with a definition of fatherhood which is firmly within the sociological tradition of placing it solely within a study of authority patterns.

In psychology, much of the literature has centred on the impact of fathers on the development of children, especially of girls. Sue Sharpe (1994) has recently analysed the often-complex relationship between fathers and daughters, which has previously been a neglected subject. It was often argued by some psychologists that so-called 'high-dominance' or successful women had identified with their father rather than their mother through childhood. Famous examples of this pattern are Florence Nightingale, and of course, Margaret Thatcher who even omitted any mention of her mother in her entry in *Who's Who*.

Anthropology, on the other hand, gives examples of other cultures where the role of the father is given very different definitions from that in Western societies. In some tribes a man is said to give birth in the same way as a woman and men will clutch their stomachs and roll in agony on the ground when their child is being born (Mead, 1950). One famous example from this study is that when describing a man, others talked of him as being prematurely aged 'because he has had many children'. There are other examples of men putting a child to their nipples and 'feeding' them.

But historically and socially in Western cultures, fatherhood tended to be a peripheral state which only became central in studies of power and authority but not in studies of childhood development or bonding. According to Nicolson (1993) in clear contrast to mothers, fathers are represented as adding positive ingredients to the beleaguered and insufficient mother–child relationship. She quotes Parke (1981), who describes fathers' involvement as improving children's intellectual and social capacities.

It is only in the past two decades that the father's role in pregnancy and childbirth has entered into any recognition in midwifery practice. There is no doubt that becoming a father is a major life event and even though the physical effects are less, the transition to a new role is stressful, traumatic and generally not acknowledged (Kitzinger, 1980).

Bedford and Johnson (1988) argue that as a result of industrialisation and urbanisation fathers spent more time working away from home and as a result woman 'took over' child-rearing and the home whilst the father's domain became work. These authors believe that as society became more complex and industrialised, the role of institutions became more important and childbirth moved to hospital. They claim that this has left men isolated and reluctant to become emotionally committed to childbearing. They argue that the father must be reinstated in birth so as to take an active role in childbirth and child-rearing. They believe that men who are supportive of their wives enable them to become better [*sic*] mothers.

Summersgill (1993) argues that fathers lost their links with couvade behaviours when birth moved from home to hospital. Couvade is a custom amongst some peoples by which a father retires to bed at the birth of his child as if in labour himself. He believes that it is only recently that social scientists have rediscovered fathers and fatherhood but that current literature tends to focus on the clinical contexts where fathers can assist with labour and delivery. He argues that the social dimensions surrounding pregnancy and birth and the needs of fathers have been ignored. He explains that fathers see hospitals 'as a culturally alien environment, where he encounters a mass of nameless, faceless experts using a 'foreign' language, together with a barrage of technological gadgets'.

He describes the problems of partners being taken away, being ignored by midwives and being made to feel a stranger or an outsider in what is 'women's business'. He believes that fathers are marginalised and excluded from all decision making during childbirth. There is a down side to men's intimate involvement with the birth process. O'Driscoll (1994) describes problems uncovered during psychosexual therapy that can be traced back to witnessing birth. She claims that assumptions about the place of men at the delivery and their involvement in childbirth have not been adequately researched. She states that evidence from Relate (formerly Marriage Guidance) indicates that relationship problems following childbirth are not unusual and that many men do not always find it easy to see the maternal role as complementing the role of lover, they are more likely to see the roles as conflicting. She argues that men need to fulfil a role that defines fathering skills as distinct from mothering skills, which should be considered as equally important.

In a study by Malcolm Macmillan of the Royal College of Midwives (Reid, 1994) it was demonstrated, somewhat surprisingly, that despite the myths and anecdotes, 88 per cent of new fathers did not feel pressurised to be present at the birth of their child. This extensive survey of 441 men in 217 locations found that 98 per cent of men planned to be present, 18 per cent helped to cut the cord, and 85 per cent of men had watched their babies being born. The study indicated men felt confused and ill-informed immediately after the birth. He argues that the compulsion should be removed and that couples themselves should decide. It is certainly true that partners are now expected to attend the birth and are judged as somewhat inadequate if they do not. Marjorie Tew (1995) argues that men, as obstetricians, are generally excluded from participating in normal birth, this is women's work (that of the midwife) where men's involvement is marginal. Tew takes this belief a stage further and uses it to explain another theory of the medicalisation of childbirth.

In describing the male takeover of birth, she suggests that the motives for men becoming involved in maternity care may arise from the deep fantasy of a strong man rescuing the weak women from distress and danger. She suggests that men who have initiated the process at conception resent, at least subconsciously, their subsequent exclusion and their implied inferiority. She suggests anthropologists have interpreted this resentment in male obstetricians who need to reassert their superiority over women when their bodies fail to perform adequately. She argues that male superiority is reasserted most emphatically when, during a Caesarian section, he cuts open the womb and extracts the baby without any assistance from the mother. She suggests an even more cynical theory of male dominance of childbirth as a fundamental counter-attack on women's struggle for political and economic equality. She says, 'Cynics see this as a salutary demonstration that inroads into man's territory have been accompanied by the surrender of her own, woman's territory – a universal acknowledgement of her essential subservience,' (Marjorie Tew, 1995). Fatherhood, like motherhood, is a complex state.

Case Study 5.1   Unhappiness following childbirth

Susan is married to David, a builder, and they own their home which they are in the process of renovating. Susan had hoped that the new bathroom would have been installed by the time her son was born but he arrived a little early. David works long hours, especially in the summer months and has worked even more hours since the baby was born. He does little about the house as he sees his main tasks as finishing the bathroom and earning enough money to compensate for the loss of Susan's earnings as a cashier. Although they have been married for one year they have both found the transition to parenthood stressful and difficult. David sleeps on the sofa so as not to disturb his wife or the baby. He believes that Susan is tense and the mess in the house is getting her down. Susan's mother died six months ago and she has no contact with her father. Her father lost touch after his divorce when Susan was 10 years old.

Susan's baby was born four weeks ago. She had a long labour, an ineffective epidural anaesthetic and a forceps delivery. She feels little joy in her new status as a mother and weeps openly. When she is encouraged to talk she explains that she felt trapped during labour and was unable to escape the tubes, wires and monitors and now she feels trapped by her son, Thomas.

She explains to the midwife who is visiting her that she is afraid to leave the house or even go to the toilet in case anyone steals her son. Then she admits quietly it might be all right or even better if she did not have a son. The baby is well cared for but Susan does not appear to look at him directly. Between the tears and the sighs she explains that she feels inadequate and unable to cope. She feels that she does not love Thomas enough and is worried by the rash on his face. She says she feels tired all the time and is not eating properly. Although she is tired most of the day she has difficulty in going to sleep.

■ Questions and discussion points

- Susan is clearly very unhappy and distressed. What 'illness' is she suffering from?
- What social factors might be contributing to her unhappiness?
- Are there any other factors in the case study which may be influencing Susan's health?
- What help can the midwife offer to Susan? What other agencies may contribute to her care?
- Would Susan be described as 'good' mother or a 'bad' mother? Justify your answer.

Key points

- Motherhood has long been culturally assumed to be the state to which all 'natural women' aspire – in other words all women want children.
- Motherhood is socially defined, limited and constructed and is not the natural state of women.
- Changes in social policy have had the effect of raising the status of women as mothers and subjecting them to state surveillance, supervision and intervention.
- Ideologies defining women's place as in the home have been reflected in state policies.
- Post-natal depression is not simply a physical illness with a physical cause. For many women adjusting to motherhood is stressful and depressing.
- Good and bad mothers are defined by society and not by their differing skills and talents.
- Bonding is a myth which emphasises the need for a relationship to be established between mothers and children at birth. It assumes incorrectly that good mothers are those who have bonded with their children and have well-developed maternal instinct. Bad mothers are deviants who have not bonded and are lacking in maternal instinct.
- In Western cultures fathers and fatherhood have not been studied in great depth.
- The transition to fatherhood is less well recognised in the literature than the transition to motherhood.

PART II

Social Policy, Women and Professionalisation

Part II

Chapter 6

Social policy, family and community

The women whom midwives meet in their day-to-day working lives are part of a new and rapidly changing environment. Child-bearing women live in the world shaped by social policy. In this chapter we will discover how social policy is framed and how government decisions impact on the lives of women and their families. The midwife who works in a hospital or in the community, or both, must be aware of the issues and their implications for the lives of women. A midwife should be able to understand the complexities of social policy, its driving forces and effects and be able to give women appropriate advice. Where the advice is complex she should know where to turn for help. It is crucial therefore that midwives understand the effects of policies on women's lives and subsequently on their own practice.

As we discussed in Chapter 3, sociologists view structures such as 'the family' and 'community' as social phenomena which contain constructed meanings within a specific society and culture. Social-policy writers, however, also focus upon the role of government legislation as the channel by which these meanings become institutionalised within the framing and enactment of social policies. Social policies affect everyone, they form the basis of our commonsense reality and lived experiences. Policies on health, housing and education are fundamental to people's life-chances and frame their expectations and beliefs.

Policies are framed by political parties when in power and represent the basic beliefs and ideals of different political philosophies. Policies are also framed within a surrounding domestic economic reality and affected by external factors such as international events and global development.

In Britain, the role of the state in policies on the family and the construction of a 'model' family by social legislation has been crucial. Fundamental to this model has been the way in which gender roles have been institutionalised within health and social welfare legislation. Far from remaining a cultural category, gender became the base structure upon which 'the family' was constructed by policies.

This chapter will focus upon an overview of the construction and application of the model family in social policies in Britain during this century and especially since the founding of the welfare state after 1945. As we have seen in Chapter 4, the social role of women is inextricably bound up with definitions of 'the family' and we will be concentrating on the specific effect of social policies on women in the next chapter.

Earlier chapters have explored the issue of the *social construct* of gender roles and family relationships, the main focus of this chapter is to look at the role of the state in the institutionalisation and the naturalisation of these structures. There are two principal themes in this exploration:

1. the intervention by the state into the so-called 'private' sphere of personal relationships with legislation on marriage and divorce in the formation of the model family;
2. the 'public' nature of the relationship between the state and 'the family' in the care and protection of children and other vulnerable groups.

The relationship between the state and children has altered enormously during the twentieth century with the state taking on a protective as well as custodial role and policies on 'community care' appear to place responsibility for vulnerable family members back within the sphere of 'the family' itself. This leads us to pose the question of the *authority* of the state as regards to family life: is 'the family' a construction of social policies ?

■ 'The family' in social policy

This division of family life into 'private' and 'public' spheres is highly questionable, for throughout this century the state has increasingly intervened in the personal lives of people and has brought 'the family' into the forefront of public policies and political rhetoric and ideology.

Although Britain does not have a Ministry for the Family as such, nevertheless ideas of what constitutes a family and the responsibility of the state in the protection of 'family life and values' permeate policies on health, housing and education as well as child protection and child care, employment and equal opportunities. Policies on 'the family' have also become connected in recent years with policies on that other structure – 'the community'. At present (1995) all the main political parties in Britain have taken ideas of 'the family' and 'community' and placed them at the centre of debate and projected policies. In the USA too, political rhetoric on 'family values' and the 'sanctity of family life' have ceased to be the sole property of the right wing (Abbott and Wallace, 1992) and have become a part of mainstream debate.

When the phrase 'the traditional family' is used in popular and political discourse it nearly always signifies the nuclear family living in close contact with other relations and based upon authority structures which reflect gender roles. How did this model become so firmly embedded in our welfare system ? It is argued by many writers (Colwill, 1994; Van Every,

1992; Riley, 1984) that the Beveridge Plan (1942), which laid the basis for the structure of health and welfare policies in post-war Britain, was based upon this specific definition of 'the family'. It consisted of a *male breadwinner* and a *female unpaid carer* within a *married* relationship with the financial responsibility for wife and children being that of the man and the care of children and elderly or sick relatives being that of the woman. These strictly demarcated roles were written into the policies on social security, national insurance, health care, education, employment, child care and housing and continue to form a part of our welfare provision today. As Elizabeth Wilson (1977) has written 'the welfare state is, above all, a set of ideas'. The Beveridge Plan in many ways reflected the dominant ideas of the time on the 'naturalness' of gender roles and of the role of men as wage-earners and women as mothers and carers who were financially dependent upon the male wage-earner. This was not merely an idea, it formed the structure of the welfare benefit system. For centuries the law had assumed that parents were responsible for children, husbands for wives and adult children for aged parents, but what made the Beveridge proposals significant was that they institutionalised within a social welfare system the legislative change of responsibility from extended family relationships to those of the nuclear family with a man at its head (Crowther, 1982).

Beveridge set out a dual insurance system within which married women would become wholly dependent upon their husbands' National Insurance contributions for any benefits. Marriage, it was assumed, would be a woman's 'sole occupation'. As the Report stated;

> During marriage most women will not be gainfully employed. The small minority of women who undertake paid employment require special treatment differing from that of a single woman. (Beveridge, 1942, p. 50)

Ironically, even at the time that the National Insurance Act was passed in 1946 the number of married women in the workforce was actually increasing. This trend was unstoppable, and despite the 'model' encapsulated in the Beveridge Report, married women's involvement in the external world of employment never slowed.

But the organisation and application of the male earner female dependent relationship of the family continues to underpin many areas of social security, employment, child care and taxation until the present day. This pattern is still often idealised as a 'norm' against which other forms of family structures or relationships are seen as somehow 'deviant'.

We now look in more detail at the specific policies which have constructed, reinforced and at times, appear to have contradicted this model. First, the policies on the more 'private' sphere of family relationships: how have these been modelled by social policies ?

■ Policies on marriage and divorce

One of the most important ways in which 'the family' was created was by the function of the legitimation of children within a relationship. Initially this was only of importance in terms of inheritance for the rich, but throughout the eighteenth and nineteenth centuries, marriage became increasingly essential to many aspects of social life.

Social policies at specific historical periods act both to encourage marriage and to discourage or even outlaw divorce, and at other times appear to have the opposite effect. But for the past century, the main influence on the availability of both marriage and divorce has been the law, with the once-powerful influence of religion decreasing.

For the majority of the population before the early nineteenth century, formal marriage sanctioned by the Church of England was a relatively minor occurrence for the urban and rural working class. John Gillis (1985) has recorded the popularity of 'little weddings' among various communities, these being informal ceremonies or rituals whereby a couple signified to their neighbours the stability of their relationship and the legitimacy of their children. Even today, the category of a 'common law' spouse remains a legally recognised status. But the state did not recognise marriages performed in non-conformist churches and chapels (to which the majority of the working class belonged) until the Civil Marriage Act of 1836, and secular State marriages did not exist until 1853.

During the early twentieth century the practice of official marriage became more and more common and it was increasingly seen as a means of access to certain economic and social benefits. Proof of marriage by the production of 'lines' was required before the payment of allowances to dependents during the First World War and widows of servicemen also had to provide proof of their status. The allocation of philanthropic and public housing was also dependent upon a marriage certificate as a proof of respectability. The age of consent was set at 16 in 1877 (it was previously 14), but *paternal* permission (unless mother was a widow) was required for marriages to take place between people under the age of 21. The increasing stress upon marriage as not only desirable but essential for access to citizenship rights was especially important for women, as we shall see in the next chapter.

After the Second World War, marriage reached a peak of popularity among working-class people and the occasion of the Church wedding set the seal of respectability (Fletcher, 1962). In 1963, only one parent's permission and not necessarily that of the father, was required for marriages under the age of 21 and the age at which marriages could be contracted without parental consent was lowered to 18 in 1969 to be congruent with the new voting age.

By the 1980s, however, marriage appeared to have lost some of its appeal. The Marriage Act of 1994 can be seen as an attempt to popularise marriages by allowing them to be performed in any premises which had the approval of the Local Authority. One of the first performed under this Act was at a football stadium.

For most of the twentieth century, however, the increasing availability and the necessity of marriage to gain access to welfare benefits contrasted with the stigmatisation of unmarried motherhood and the legal cost, complexity and stigma of gaining a divorce.

Historically, divorce was only available to a minute minority whose case had to be debated in Parliament (Stone, 1990). The Divorce Act of 1857 removed it from the jurisdiction of the Church and placed divorce within a legal framework with the setting-up of the Court for Divorce and Matrimonial Matters. It remained expensive and only the wealthier middle classes could consider taking this step. The Church of England would not remarry the 'guilty party' and there was no concept of 'mutual guilt' and in the case of adultery (even if mutual) only that of the wife counted. From then to the present day, divorce settlements became seen as the responsibility of the legal profession and (unlike marriage) are not given any religious connotations.

Despite this secularisation of divorce, it remained a social stigma and a scandal and especially for women it spelt the end of entry to respectable society. The reasons for which a divorce could be gained differed between men and women. Adultery could be the sole reason for a man's claim but for women, their husband's adultery had to be accompanied by other factors such as cruelty, insanity or alcoholism. It was not until the Infants Custody Act of 1925, that married women became legal guardians of their legitimate children. Until as late as the 1960s, women almost invariably lost custody of their children after a divorce.

Slowly throughout the twentieth century, access to divorce was widened, both in respect of the accepted causes and the financial cost. The Divorce Act of 1923 gave wives the right to divorce for adultery only on the same basis as men. The Matrimonial Causes Act of 1937 added desertion of three years to the permissible causes but the marriage had to be of five years duration. The level of divorce rose rapidly in the following years almost doubling between 1937 and 1939.

The biggest boost to the availability of divorce for the mass of the population came with the Legal Aid Act of 1949. This meant that the cost of divorce could be underwritten and so it became much more widely accessible to lower income groups. After both wars, the number of divorces rose with the majority of cases being brought by husbands in respect of wives' adultery and desertion. Throughout the 1950s and 1960s, divorce was still feared by many women and it was men who were the majority of plaintiffs. The idea of 'guilt' was very strong in divorce legislation with the identity of the 'guilty party' being bestowed upon errant wives and husbands. Despite its increasing occurrence among film stars, famous personalities and the wealthy, divorce retained its stigma. Sir

Antony Eden was the first divorced man to become Prime Minister in 1953 and as late as the 1960s divorced people were not admitted to the Royal Enclosure at Ascot.

This period of restriction and puritanical social mores ended with the Divorce Reform Act 1969, which came into effect in 1971. This legislation opened the gates to divorce within a specific period of time and removed the legal requirement of 'proving guilt'. Divorce by consent of the two people was all that was needed with the 'irretrievable breakdown of marriage' as the basic factor. People could be divorced even without their consent after a period of seven years' separation; this led to great controversy, especially from religious groups. This legislation changed the face of marriage and divorce in Britain. Within the first year, the divorce rate doubled, owing to the tremendous backlog of marriages that had in fact ended in the previous years. The custody of children became a matter for the family courts and women gained the majority of custody cases. After this Act, the divorce rate doubled and women also became the majority plaintiffs (by 1990 over 75 per cent of cases were brought by women).

In 1984 the Matrimonial and Family Proceedings Act further eroded the concept of marriage as a 'sole occupation for life' with the entitlement to maintenance being withdrawn from ex-wives who had no children and were aged under 30. It also reduced the length of separation by which a marriage could be dissolved without the agreement of both partners, from seven to five years, and allowed couples to petition for divorce after one year rather than three years of marriage. Most importantly, it introduced the idea of the 'clean break' into divorce settlements with the objective of encouraging women to become more self-sufficient.

Under the Children Act (1989) if a divorced woman remarries she is no longer entitled to any maintenance from her ex-husband but he continues to be liable for child maintenance.

There was much discussion in the early 1990s on the need for Divorce Law Reform, with the suggestions that divorce be made more difficult to obtain and that courts should have the right to refuse to grant one if economic hardship to one of the parties was deemed to be likely. In 1995, after much party political controversy, Lord Mackay's White Paper on divorce reform was published. It would remove the necessity to prove 'fault' in a marriage but would compel the couple to undergo a year's mediation and to encourage them to negotiate their own settlements without the services of a lawyer. The delay of a year has been seen as an attempt to end so-called 'quickie' divorces. There was also a government proposal that courts should take pension rights into consideration when splitting the assets gained through marriage. This may entitle divorced women to claim a portion of their ex-husband's pension on retirement.

Because of social legislation in the 1960s and 1970s, both marriage and divorce became easier to obtain. But despite this change in one area of social policy, the *model* of 'the family' remained ideologically intact.

The Beveridge reforms made no specific allowance for divorced wives/mothers or for unmarried mothers. It was assumed that these would be a small minority and although originally Beveridge had proposed the payment of an 'end-of-marriage allowance' to 'innocent' wives after divorce, this had been defeated. It was not until the 1980s that the growing number of women with dependent children who appeared to choose to live outside marriage gave cause for great public concern.

From the Beveridge Plan of the 1940s to the reforms of the welfare system in the 1980s and 1990s, the model of 'the family' has been modified and altered. But although the reality of social life in Britain has changed enormously in the fifty years since the Beveridge Plan, despite the increase in divorce and the decline in marriage, the state's responsibility in reinforcing certain ideas on the role and tasks of the family as a whole remain strong. The changing policies on divorce may have reflected a popular demand, and the social acceptability of lone motherhood have increased, but the welfare system as a whole continues to be conceptually based upon the male breadwinner model of the family.

■ The end of the male-breadwinner model?

Despite the continuing ideological existence and influence of the male bread winner ideal, by the 1980s its social existence was in decline. The reality in Britain today is that without women's income, poverty in households would be more widespread. It has been recently calculated (Harkness, Machin, Waldfogel, 1994), that without women's earnings poverty rates among couples would be 50 per cent higher. The typical married or cohabiting woman working part-time contributes 20 per cent of the family income and if she works full-time, more than 40 per cent (see Table 6.1).

Since the 1970s, the impact of women's earnings has been greatest in the distribution of money within low-income families. In effect, there has been a measure of 'equalisation' of income due to women's increased employment.

The pattern in Britain in 1995, is the segregation of families or households into 'dual earner' and 'no-earner' or 'work-rich' or 'work poor' as it is known. For example, in 1993 the proportion of dual earners in two-adult households was 61 per cent (a rise of 10 per cent since 1975). Conversely, the number of two-adult households with no work has tripled from 4 per cent in 1975 to over 11 per cent in 1993. Joblessness therefore tends to 'run' in households, as does dual earning. But both women and men with non-working partners have suffered the most from increasing unemployment especially in unskilled manual jobs.

Table 6.1 Proportion of net family income with and without Child Benefit contributed by women in couples, Great Britain, 1991

	Percentages of couples		
	Without Child Benefit	All income	Wife's contribution
Not dependent	12	12	45<55%
	9	10	55<100%
Dependent	20	2	Zero
	59	76	0–<45%

Sources: Adapted from National Child Development Study; Rowntree Foundation, *Social Policy Research*, 85 (November 1995).

On all measures of socio-economic standing married parents are more likely to be employed, tend to be better-educated and less likely to be on low incomes or in local authority housing, than are cohabiting or single parents (see Figure 6.1).

Women's working lives now tend to be disrupted and disadvantaged by motherhood but not by marriage. In other words, the Beveridge 'ideal' of the non-working and dependent married woman has been replaced by the non-working or part-time working mother. Dex (1987) has shown that childbirth is the single biggest factor in downward occupational mobility and rewards. After having a baby most women 'returners' enter part-time employment, sometimes with the same employer with whom they previously worked full-time. This severely handicaps promotion and pay prospects and sets the trend for the future.

The pattern of the gender-segregation of work not only by occupation but by hours worked is very striking in Britain and explains why, unlike almost all other EC countries, female unemployment is lower than that of males. Interestingly, when they do work, mothers also see as their responsibility the payment for child-care costs as the price they pay for 'choosing' to work (Brannen 1992).

The male-breadwinner model in social security policies means that female employment is seen as extra income and deductible from a family's entitlement to benefits. Couples are seen as linked and not as individual workers. Husbands are responsible for claiming benefits and these are reduced by wives' earnings. Families are therefore frequently caught in a 'poverty trap' (Morris, 1990). The trap is set because it is primarily male earnings which continue to be seen as the 'family wage'. In terms of the financial support of children however, the state has extended its responsibilities whilst still reflecting the male-breadwinner ideology.

Figure 6.1 Key facts on parents, 1992

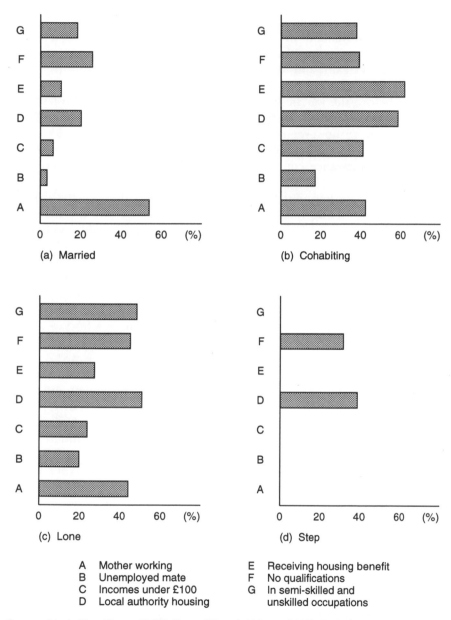

(a) Married

(b) Cohabiting

(c) Lone

(d) Step

A   Mother working
B   Unemployed mate
C   Incomes under £100
D   Local authority housing

E   Receiving housing benefit
F   No qualifications
G   In semi-skilled and
    unskilled occupations

Sources: Adapted from Kiernan (1993); *General Household Survey* (1993); *Social Security Statistics*
(1993).

■ From family allowance to family credit

The campaign for family allowances or 'wages for motherhood' was part of a larger movement in the education of mothers and the eugenic emphasis on improving the quality of the population which dominated discourses on health and welfare in the early twentieth century (see next chapter). Tax allowances for children had been paid to families of low income before the war in 1914 and during the war the income level for allowances had been raised to include some officers' families. These allowances were however payable to the wage-earner, who would in the vast majority of cases have been the husband. At the end of the war, a dependents allowance continued to be paid to ex-servicemen who were out of work.

The Family Endowment Society was formed in 1918 with the express purpose of extending this tax initiative to the payment of an allowance directly to mothers of families to combat poverty and to aid good child-rearing. It was led by Eleanor Rathbone, the Independent MP for the Combined Universities, who continued her campaign until the enactment of the policy for family allowance in 1945. There were different political and social concerns which became involved in this campaign during the inter-war years: there were those who were concerned to combat child poverty, there were feminist and women's organisations who saw it as a way of raising the status of motherhood and there were those who were anxious to halt the fall in the birth rate by encouraging maternity.

The main opposition to the idea of payment by the state to mothers for the upkeep of children came from the trade union movement and, until the Second World War, from both the Labour and Conservative parties for differing reasons. The main objection of both the Trade Unions and the Labour movement was that it would have the effect of undercutting the argument for a 'living wage' (McNichol, 1980). This phrase came to dominate wage negotiations and disputes until after the Second World War. The Unions were concerned to fight for a 'living wage' whereby a man 'could keep' his wife and children. The differentials between men's and women's pay was based upon this argument so that even if unmarried, a man could legitimately claim to have more expenses than a single woman as he had to pay for a 'phantom wife' to cook and clean for him. Men it was said, needed more money as they were expected to pay for women whether in the form of taking them out or for keeping a family. In the professions such as the civil service and teaching when equal pay was enacted, the opposition was based upon the argument that this, in fact, made single women better off than men. Once married, women were forced to resign from many jobs including the civil service, teaching, nursing and banking as it was deemed unnecessary and 'wrong' that married women should be in receipt of a wage.

Therefore for many in the Labour movement, the payment of a family allowance was viewed as a 'ploy to keep down wages ' as the Labour leader, Attlee, stated in 1938 (McNichol, 1980), although Ella Wilkinson, also a Labour MP, supported the campaign as a means of combating child poverty.

During the 1930s, with the growth in poverty and deprivation in areas of high unemployment, local authorities selected children for the receipt of certain benefits, these included free school dinners and free milk and more tax allowances were given based upon the men's wage. The demand for family allowances gained support during these years but there was great debate on how they should be funded.

During the Second World War, the Labour Party and the Trade Union movement gained in power and confidence and by 1942 showed support for a system of family allowances. In the Beveridge Report in that year the White Paper on family allowances was published. It recommended a flat-rate universal system and after much heated debate, agreed that it should be paid to the mother. Beveridge saw this payment as part of a whole package of measures on health and education and included the provision of school meals and free school milk to all. Family Allowance was paid for the first time in 1945 to the second and subsequent children only. It was decided not to pay for the first child because of cost. It was a universal payment and was the only one to which a woman was directly entitled.

During the 1950s, tax allowances for children were increased and a parent (nearly always father) could claim an allowance equal to 60 per cent of that of a single person. There was an attempt by the Labour government in the mid-1960s to claw back some of this money by reducing the tax allowance by £52 per annum for every child entitled to family allowance. This was the first attempt to move away from the universal payment and to concentrate benefit on families below the tax threshold.

In 1971, Family Income Supplement (FIS) was introduced by a Conservative administration headed by Edward Heath. It illustrated the government's commitment to switching state support from the poorest and unemployed to those in low paid work and especially the male breadwinner.

FIS was a means-tested benefit payable to families where the head of household was in full-time work with an average gross income below a certain amount. This was developed instead of upgrading the family allowances and as an interim measure before the introduction of a new system planned for 1972. In this year, the Conservative government proposed to integrate the tax and benefit systems and to introduce a system of child credits through the salary of the largest wage-earner. This was very controversial but the government fell in 1974 and the incoming Labour government also had new proposals. They proposed that the family allowance and child tax allowances should be replaced by a unified tax-free flat-rate sum payable to mothers for *every* dependent child up to

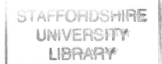

the age of 16, or 19 if in full-time education. This was also very controversial and split the cabinet as it was feared that the decrease in tax allowances in men's wages would fuel wage demands. But in 1975, the Child Benefit Bill was passed which was a non-contributory, flat-rate and universal payment for all dependent children signalling the party's ideological commitment to an egalitarian welfare system. In addition, FIS remained in place and was paid on production of an order book, usually to the mother. Families receiving FIS also kept their entitlement to other benefits such as free school dinners , housing benefit and welfare food.

The entire welfare system was destined for a radical overhaul with the election in 1979 of the New Right administration headed by Margaret Thatcher. Ideologically committed to the ideal family and 'traditional family values' as well as a belief in the emphasis on families providing for themselves and relying less on state support, the government introduced legislation which attempted to reimpose the male-breadwinner model but at the same time was forced to recognise that family structures had undergone irrevocable change.

Before 1979, maintenance paid for children by the absent father affected the dependency entitlements included in Supplementary benefit paid to the parent. In other words, if payments for children were sufficiently high, the mother would receive no payment for them under Supplementary Benefit, only for herself. This changed in 1979, and the parents' own entitlement was reduced or extinguished altogether if the father was able or willing to pay a generous maintenance payment. This meant that women were forced to become dependent on their own children via the fathers' financial generosity. In order to combat a resultant increase in child poverty, in 1981 the One-Parent Benefit was introduced which provided an extra weekly tax-free supplement to single parents in addition to child benefit. This was paid to the family, however, and not for every child. The number of lone parents receiving little or no maintenance from former spouses grew during the 1980s from 1981–2 when half of all lone parents received some maintenance to 1989 when this had fallen to less than a quarter (quoted in Millar, 1994). The takeup of all means-tested benefits varied and as can be seen in Table 6.2, it was only child benefit which could be said to have been taken up by approximately the total numbers eligible.

Although the government failed to upgrade child benefit throughout the latter part of the 1980s, it was uprated in 1991 when this became one of the first acts of the new Major administration. There is currently (1995) a political debate being conducted as to whether the Child Benefit payment should continue to be a universal one payable to all, or whether it should be targeted on groups in special need. Both the Conservative and Labour parties are engaged in the debate as to how, if a system of targeting were adopted, it could be applied. It would involve means-testing of income and many writers are concerned that this would leave

Table 6.2 Spending on and receipt of Social Security
benefits, Great Britain, 1990–1

	Recipients (000)	Amount spent (£ million)
One-Parent Benefit	760	216
Family Credit	315	4 384
Maternity Allowance	20	34
Statutory Maternity Pay	95	340
Invalid Care Allowance	25	213
Child Benefit	12 165*	4 636
	6 760**	

* Children

** Families

Source: Adapted from *Social Security: The Government's Expenditure Plans 1991–92 to 1993–4*, Cmnd 1514 (HMSO, 1991).

women even worse off than at present (Pahl, 1989). We will look at this debate in the section on women in poverty in the following chapter.

In 1985 the government published its proposals on Family Credit which was to replace FIS. Initially it was proposed that this would be paid by the employer through the man's wages. The advantage to this was that it could be withheld if the employee was on strike. This followed the 1984 miners' strike where it was claimed that Child Benefit had in fact lessened the effect of the strike on families and so had been instrumental in prolonging it. However, following lobbying by small firms who did not want the added burden of administering the payments, and by women's organisations, the government administered the payment themselves. Unlike FIS, recipients of family credit are not entitled to other benefits and it is based upon the gross rather than net income. Family Credit was put into practice in 1988: it is essentially a benefit for the 'working poor' with families who are employed for 24 hours or more per week. Take-up of this benefit is low, because for every £1 of family credit awarded this results in a loss of housing benefit /community charge of 80p, therefore the 'net worth' to the recipient is only 20p for every £1 claimed for those in rented accommodation. A study of the level of take-up of this benefit (Noble, Smith and Munby, 1992), in two areas found that single parents and those with larger families were the most likely to claim. But in one area – Oxford – the take-up rate for those eligible was less than 50 per cent, and in Oldham it was less than 70 per cent. It is apparent that many low-income and eligible families are either not claiming at all or are deterred from reapplying after an initial rejection.

Another new benefit introduced in 1988 was the Social Fund. This is a discretionary award and consists mainly of 'start-up' grants and/or loans.

Loans are by far the greatest proportion of Social Fund expenditure representing about 70 per cent but the majority of claimants apply for grants. As Table 6.3 shows single people consisting primarily of those suffering from a disability and previously in receipt of institutional care, are the group most likely to receive a 'start-up' grant with lone parents (mostly women) the second largest group. This reflects the lower priority given to families compared with those moving into community care.

Another vulnerable group which has received special consideration within the benefit system are families with a disabled child. The Family Fund was founded in 1973 and exists to provide grants to families with a severely handicapped child under the age of 16. It is a means-tested benefit and to be eligible the family must be caring for a severely handicapped child and in receipt of a low income. The fund is administered by the Joseph Rowntree Foundation on behalf of the government and since its inception has helped over 100 000 families. Grants during this period have typically covered payment for laundry equipment (67 per cent), holidays (51 per cent), transport costs (47 per cent), beds and bedding (33 per cent), and clothing (29 per cent). Applications to the Fund rose throughout the 1980s especially from parents of children aged less than one year.

There are regional variations in applications which largely follow the geographical incidence of disabling conditions. Spina bifida, congenital rubella and Downs syndrome have all declined over the past decade, probably as a result of screening and immunisation programmes, but there has been a national increase in childhood asthma and in skin complaints. The majority of asthmatics do not, however, qualify for a grant from the Fund. Other conditions such as cerebral palsy, learning disabilities and cystic fibrosis have remained relatively static. The geographical variations in the incidence of conditions and claims to the Fund, roughly mirror the 'poverty map' of Britain (see Chapter 2).

Wales and Northern Ireland have the highest recorded incidence of disability and are the largest claimants (Rowntree, 1994). Correspond-

Table 6.3 Social Fund payments, 1990

	Start up grants paid	£ share start up total (%)	Average amount (£)
2-parent families	9	9	590
Couples and other adults	7	7	325
Lone parents	32	34	644
Single people	56	49	528

Source: Adapted from Joseph Rowntree Foundation (1990); G. Stewart, 'Contribution of Social Fund in Relieving Poverty', Department of Social Administration, Lancaster, for the Rowntree Foundation (1990).

ingly, the more affluent areas of London and the south-east have relatively low rates of both disabilities and claims. The North of England has seen a rise in the incidence of disabling skin complaints among children and this has accounted for a relatively high rate of claims.

Since the Children Act in 1989, applications have risen still further. Under the Act, social services have been made responsible for maintaining a register of disabled children in their area and ensuring that their needs are met. This has resulted in a substantial increase in applications since 1990, and in 1993 alone, 34 000 families were receiving grants. Even so, the Rowntree Foundation calculate that as many as four in ten eligible families do not apply for assistance (Rowntree, 1991). The advent of both the Children Act and the move away from long-term hospitalisation has led to the increase in the numbers of very young children being granted funds.

As we have seen, the responsibility of the state to ensure that families with dependent children are supported financially has been largely accepted by different governments to the present time. The central relationship between 'the family' and the state has been based upon this responsibility and also that of the state to protect children as well as support them. In the area of child support, has the state in fact taken over the 'traditional' role of the male breadwinner ? If so, what role is there for fathers ?

■ Child support and fathers

Traditionally, the welfare state was predicated upon the belief (and institutionalised through the National Insurance system) that fathers should be financially responsible for their children. This especially applied to men living in a marital relationship with the paternity of the children accepted as his own. Historically, the father of one or more illegitimate children could be forced to assume a measure of financial responsibility through an order made against him. In 1872, a law was passed requiring a father to pay 5 shillings a week towards the upkeep of the child and this was extended in 1918 to the sum of 10 shillings per week. But in order to claim this money a woman had to 'prove' paternity and this was often such a long, complex and often humiliating experience that many did not attempt it. Fathers had no claim on their illegitimate children but these children were judged to be the responsibility of the mother and, if all else failed, the Poor Law.

Marriage, on the other hand, endowed husbands and fathers with authority over their children and also gave them strict duties to support them. With the increase in divorce and single motherhood from the 1970s, the reliance on the 'male breadwinner' which was always subject to individual variations, appeared to break down altogether. The payment of maintenance by divorced husbands declined in numbers throughout the 1980s and of the mothers who were 'never married' by 1991 only 1 in 7 was receiving any payment from the father (Millar, 1994). After the Matrimonial Proceedings Act of 1984 had introduced the concept of 'the clean break' into divorce settlements, this often resulted in a man signing over the family house to his ex-wife (with the mortgage payments often then becoming the responsibility of the DHSS) as payment in lieu of continuous maintenance. These factors posed great financial problems for the state as despite the government's wish to cut back on benefit payments and to end dependency on benefits, the actual costs were rising (See Figure 6.2). The other reason for this growth in female 'dependency' on the state, was the increasing number of mothers who never married. The picture was further complicated by the fact that men were far more likely than women to remarry after divorce and so begin a second family.

Political concern over the 'flight of the fathers' reached a crescendo by 1990. Suddenly, it was fatherhood rather than motherhood which moved to the top of the political agenda. Peter Lilley, the then Minister for Social Security, stated in 1994; 'The state has made mothers dependent and fathers redundant'. In 1995, John Redwood a leading Conservative right-wing politician, argued that young single mothers should be urged to give up their babies for adoption. Much of the criticism voiced over the rise in welfare payments was founded on the fact that many men failed to support their children and so turned over their responsibilities to the state.

Much of the concern over the role of men stemmed from the writing of an American radical conservative theorist, Charles Murray. Murray (1990),

Figure 6.2   Numbers of lone parents* on Income
Support, all ages, 1979 and 1994/5

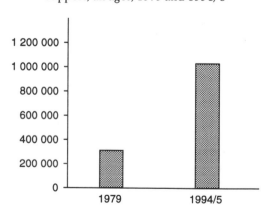

* Never married, divorced, separated or widowed.

Source: Indepenedent (15 August 1995). Reproduced by permission.

writing of the situation among inner-city black population in the USA, argued that it was because of the increase in state benefits and the decline in the stigmatisation of unmarried motherhood that fathers were now deemed redundant. He went on to argue that this was the single biggest cause of crime and violence and that single mothers and their unsupported children now formed a new 'underclass'. This 'underclass' theory was taken up in the British context by sociologists Norman Dennis and George Erdos (1993), who, writing against the background of the Meadow Well Estate riots on Tyneside in 1991, also put forward the view that it was men's lives which had been uprooted by economic depression and feminist gains made through the intervention of the state. Men, he argued had lost their role as responsible fathers and breadwinners and that the rise in young male crime and deviancy was the direct result of the feminist objective of freeing women from the ties of dependency within the traditional family. These views found much support among both Conservatives and traditional Labour supporters. Beatrix Campbell (1993) gave a feminist analysis to the breakdown in family structures and the increase in male crime when she argued that it was essentially a crisis of masculinity which was being addressed in a period of economic decline and high unemployment. Women, she argued, were rejecting dependency on individual men who are unemployed and unreliable and preferred dependence on the state. Hilary Graham in her research on unsupported mothers also argued that many women were better-off on state support even if their actual income had fallen, as it gave them control over all the finances. The moral panic over fatherhood meant that the British government either had to adopt an alternative model of welfare provision or attempt to reinforce the strong male-breadwinner model which had crumbled. It chose the latter.

In 1991, a report entitled *Children Come First* was published which contained the results of limited research on absent fathers and which showed that the majority were more likely to be unemployed or of a lower income than the general male population. But legislation in Australia which had been introduced to combat poverty among single mothers had proved a success. So in 1991 the Child Support Act was introduced in Britain and proved immediately controversial. Under this Act, single parents who were receiving no maintenance from the absent 'parent' were required to name the (father) so that the *Child Support Agency* could contact (him) for maintenance payments. There were two important issues here; first, the generic word 'parent' was used throughout the Act although in 99 per cent of cases it was absent fathers who were pursued, second, women were required to name a person for payment but their actual income was not going to be increased. Even more controversially, the Child Support Agency was given a target for savings by the Government, and this encouraged them, it was alleged by opponents, to pursue men who were 'soft targets'. It was true that it tended to be men who were already paying some maintenance to ex-wives and families who appeared to be in the majority of those called to account by the Agency. Furthermore, and even more controversially, previous Court rulings on 'clean break' divorce settlements were overturned and many men, some with second families, were faced with spiralling demands for maintenance.

Public opinion appeared at first, to be fully supportive of the idea behind the Act, to make fathers financially accountable for their children and to cut the burden on the taxpayer, but this support led to unease after a series of media reports on some personal tragedies. Men were said to have committed suicide when faced with demands from the Agency and pressure groups were formed of men and their second families who carried out many public demonstrations against the Act during 1992 and 1993.

In 1995, the Government published a White paper *Improving Child Support* which announced alterations and changes to the original proposals. The main change was that the 'carer' parent who was in work and not on benefits would not have recourse to the Agency after 1996, but they would still have to go to court for a maintenance judgement. Other changes included a limit of 30 per cent of normal net income to be payable in maintenance, housing costs and travel-to-work costs allowed to 'second' families. As from 1997, parents with the care of children, who are on income support or job-seekers allowance, will be able to build up a 'maintenance credit' from that clawed back by the Treasury, up to £1000, which will be payable as a lump sum when they start work. This is to offset some of the disadvantages of coming off benefit such as the loss of free school milk and dental care.

These changes had many critics. The Government was accused of bowing to the pressure from men who had abdicated their responsibilities and also of doing nothing to relieve child poverty. It also reinforced people's belief that the real motivation behind the Act was to save the Treasury money by getting people off benefit and into work. So the efforts by the State to force absent 'fathers' to pay adequately for child support remained as controversial as ever.

Why had the scheme been a success in Australia and a relative failure in Britain? The main reason, argue Millar and Whiteford (1993), is that the motivation behind the Act differed in the two countries. In Australia, it was part of a package of measures to combat poverty, in Britain it was seen primarily as a money-saving exercise promoted by the Treasury. Recipients of increased maintenance gained financially in Australia whereas in Britain they appeared to be no better-off. Finally, the legislation in Australia was phased-in over a long period of time with adequate advance warning given, and was not retrospective as in Britain. In Australia it had gained public support from most quarters, unlike the situation in Britain where many groups had opposed its introduction.

The Child Support Act can be seen as an attempt to reinforce the authority and responsibility of the male breadwinner by replacing female dependency on the state with dependency on the individual male. The interests of children themselves also formed an important shift in policies on child care and child protection.

■ Child care and child protection

Social policies on child care, carry two different interpretations:

1. the provision of actual 'hands-on' daily care and supervision of young pre-school children;
2. the removal of children from their families into the care of local authorities.

The first type of policy will be dealt with in the following chapter when we review the state and private provision of child care in Britain since the war.

The second type was the basis of social work with children from the 1970s until the Children Act 1989. During the 1970s increasing numbers of children were being removed compulsorily from parental care into the auspices of council homes. After much criticism during the early 1980s, a new model of child care was sought which shifted the emphasis of social work on to a 'more professionalised model of good child care, emphasising partnership, family support, maintaining links and the aim of returning children to their family of origin' (Langan, 1993, p. 154).

During the 1980s there had been a deluge of media publicity surrounding child abuse cases and child deaths. As Allen Cochrane (1993) has argued, in the 1970s and early 1980s most of the adverse publicity concerned the ineptness of social workers who failed to remove into care a child who was subsequently killed within the family. The late 1980s saw public criticism of social workers as being too anxious to remove children from their families after suspected child abuse. The Cleveland Inquiry in 1987 was probably the most significant in its effect on the subsequent legislation, but there were other Inquiries into 'ritual' and 'satanic' abuse during this period. Altogether there were eighteen official inquiries into child abuse during the 1980s. The outcome of this activity was the acceptance by the government of the need to set a structure and 'standards for professional relationships to parents and children [as] in the Cleveland report' (DoH, 1991, p. 111).

The Children Act 1989, which was implemented in 1991, was the legislative result of all the previous concerns with professional practice and the parental responsibilities towards children. The key messages of the Act are: first, that children are best cared for within their own families; second, that the interests of the child are paramount, and third, that these objectives can best be attained through a partnership between the social services and families of children 'in need'. The accommodation and care of disabled children up to the age of 18, including the assessment, provision of services, and the integration of services with those of other children in need, became under the Act, the responsibility of local authorities and not the Health Service (as for adults). The role of parents is heavily emphasised in the Act; *parental responsibility* was a new term which covered all the rights, powers and duties of parents and gave this to the State only via a court judgement. Nick Allen (1991) argues that this represented a new concept which was similar to that of legal custody. Married parents shared equal responsibility *even after divorce*, unmarried fathers had no automatic responsibility but could apply for a measure and an unmarried couple could enter a written agreement regarding parental rights and responsibilities. After divorce, one person was to be designated as the *caring* parent with a *residence order*, in the event of the possible death of the caring parent a guardian (possibly grandparent or other friend or relation) could be appointed to share care on a joint basis with the other parent. The main aim of the Act was to strengthen the continuing role of 'parenting' even after the end of a marriage.

There have been critics of the wording and orientation of the Act. Miriam David (1989) has argued that the wording of 'parental responsibility' is not gender-blind but a reinforcement of the assumption that it is mothers who will be the 'caring' parent and the need to 'co-parent' after divorce will be strongly felt by them for financial reasons (see Child Support Act). She also questions the emphasis on 'the family' and argues that policies only become applicable after family breakdown thus strengthening the private arena of family life. The emphasis on a specific model of ' the family' in the consciousness and practice of social work has been challenged by many writers (Clarke, 1993, pp. 107–9). There is a fear that only a heterosexual nuclear and preferably white family with a man at the head really conforms to the model with any other formations seen as 'deviant'.

But what the Children Act represented was the idea that children although 'belonging' to parents whilst in a marriage needed to be safeguarded after divorce and that it was the responsibility of the State to oversee and ensure that this happened. Likewise, the state takes the responsibility for children who for one reason or another need care away from their own homes.

■ Adoption and fostering

In 1991, approximately 75 000 children in the UK were being cared for by local authorities (see Figure 6.3). The majority of children are mainly from low-income working-class families in deprived inner city areas (Thoburn, 1994). Among ethnic minorities, Asian children are underrepresented and children of Caribbean or African parentage are overrepresented among children in care. Children of 'mixed race' are more likely than either black or white children to be placed in care. The 'breakdown in family' is the most cited reason given (69 per cent of cases) with the behaviour of the child him/herself as the second most common reason (25 per cent of cases). Interestingly, poverty, bad housing or material need are rarely mentioned by social workers in this regard. Children from single-parent families are at a greater risk of coming into care and also those from 'reconstituted' families. In 1990, over 4 000 children entered care because of the ill-health – mainly mental health – of their parent or guardian.

Figure 6.3 Children in care, admissions to care and children removed to a place of safety, England and Wales, 1981–91

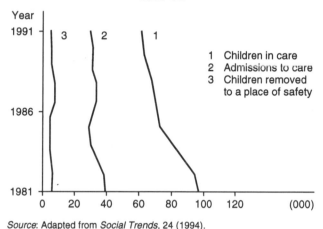

Source: Adapted from *Social Trends*, 24 (1994).

There have been two main means of supplying a family structure to children with either long-term or short-term needs, adoption and fostering. The number of children available for adoption has fallen dramatically in recent years, from 25 000 adoptions in 1968 to just 9 000 in 1986 (Kahan, 1989). As is discussed in Chapter 5, the change in society's attitudes to single motherhood and the legalisation of abortion has meant that the pool of babies previously deemed suitable for adoption has all but disappeared. The popular demand for 'white, healthy babies' cannot be met and this has led in recent years to the increase in the adoption of babies from countries such as Romania and Bosnia, sometimes accompanied by bad publicity and discouraged by social services and children's organisations.

Legal adoption was originally intended to aid childless couples in giving a 'fresh start' to a child. For this reason the adoption was kept a secret and hedged around with silence and almost shame. The 1949 Act allowed adopters to remain anonymous in court proceedings so that they could not be traced by the natural parents in future years. This attitude remained officially until the 1975 Act. The Houghton Committee which began work in 1969, saw access to birth information as a right and this was supported by many organisations. The move to 'open' adoption underpinned the Children Act of 1975 when the adopted person's right to their birth records became law. A tracing and counselling service is now offered by all local authorities and social services.

In order to qualify as adoptive parents, people have to undergo stringent interviews and home visits. The model of the ideal family for adoption purposes has been criticised by many. It is argued that the model of the white heterosexual family headed by a man is far too narrow a definition of suitability. People such as lesbians or gay men who do not 'fit' the model find it very difficult to adopt or even foster a child. The Adoption Act of 1976 stipulates that only married couples or single people can apply to adopt a child (Clarke, 1993).

An issue which has become very important in recent years is that of transracial adoption. During the 1960s it was common practice to place black children with white families. Black infants were not 'hard to place' in the absence of same-race children (Thoburn, 1994). But in the 1980s research showed that black children brought up by white parents failed to develop a positive cultural or racial identity (Ahmad, 1989). It was often said that there were not sufficient numbers of black families who were willing to adopt or foster, but when the New Black Families Unit opened in 1986 it received fifty applications in the first four months (Ahmad, 1989).

The normal practice now is 'black families for black children' and the Children Act stipulates that local authorities must pay heed to 'the child's religious persuasion, racial origin and cultural and linguistic background' (Sec.22, 5, c).

Fostering, unlike adoption, is seen as a short-term or emergency measure. Although foster care can be long-term and seen as permanent by those involved, fostering is regarded officially as a short-term measure. Fostering 'with a view to adoption' has almost ceased to exist in Britain although fostering by relatives is relatively common and recent research has shown that this is the most stable form of fostering (HMSO, 1991). Foster-parents provide a service for social services by mainly fostering abused or 'in need' children on an emergency basis or supplying long-term care for those unable or unlikely to return home. Berridge and Cleaver (1987) found that the breakdown rate in long-term fostering was between 20 and 40 per cent over five years.

In 1989, a study entitled Child Care Now (Rowe *et al.*) reported that children over 11 years old were most likely to be in residential care (62 per cent) compared with only 6 per cent of children under 4 years old. Children under 4 were most likely to be in foster homes (77 per cent) compared with only 15 per cent of children above the age of 11.

The Children Act which since 1989 has emphasised working with parents to keep families together and to prevent intervention, has had the effect of reducing the number of children now being placed in care (Figure.6.3).

This pattern of non-institutionalised care has also been extended to other vulnerable groups.

■ Community care

The idea of placing the care of certain social groups, especially people with a learning disability or mental illness, outside formal institutions and into 'the community' was proposed by a government Health Minister (Enoch Powell) as early as 1961. Even earlier than that, the Guillebaud Committee had made out a case for a policy of community-based care in 1956 (Baggott, 1994). Following a series of publicised scandals involving the treatment of mental patients in certain long-stay institutions during the 1960s, support for a policy of de-hospitalisation for mental patients grew. The developments in drugs during this time also made the treatment and control of certain mental illnesses through medication feasible and more economic than long hospital stays. During the 1970s both Labour and Conservative governments attempted to redirect scarce resources within the Health service towards the so-called 'Cinderella' services for the frail elderly and people with a mental handicap and mental health problems.

But the Thatcher administration during the 1980s showed the most determination to shift the balance of health care from the hospital-based services to the community. This was part of a whole set of reforms to the Health Service which were enacted during the 1980s (see Chapter 7) and which aimed to bring market principles, managerial control, and an extension of the role of the voluntary sector and family in the provision of care within the Health Service.

The Griffiths Review 1988 which was commissioned by the government set out three guides for the implementation of such a policy:

1. that services should be provided early to people who needed them most;
2. that people should have more choice and a say in their own care,
3. that people should be cared for wherever possible in their own homes and not referred for residential or nursing home and hospital care if it could be avoided.

It also argued that the NHS was inadequate, badly managed and lacked the vision to bring about change.

The organisation of community care was to be delegated to local authorities who would be responsible for the planning, assessing and provision of care in the locality. Probably the most controversial suggestion was that health care was to be separated from social care and that the overall responsibility for the organisation and management of care was to be given to the Social Services. Local managers of care from the Social Services were to carry out the assessment of people and to plan individual care packages tailored to individual needs. This meant that a far closer working relationship between health-care workers · such as district nurses, health visitors, community psychiatric nurses and GPs and social workers was needed than had previously existed. Local authorities and not central Social Services were to be made responsible for the allocation of funds for community care, including the payment of fees in residential homes. Central government would continue to allocate funds to local authorities but these would not be 'ring-fenced' – that is reserved for community care plans – but would represent a static total amount. Many local authorities were worried that the funds would not be sufficient to pay for the needs for community-based care and many Health Authorities were opposed to the whole idea of transferring care from hospital to community-based services.

The National Health Service and Community Care Act 1990 was passed and then was delayed before implementation in 1993. The delay enabled the government to make alterations to the original proposal, the most important of which was the increase in funding. From April 1993, local authorities have received a 'ring-fenced' payment known as the 'Special Transitional Grant' which is for three years duration to enable community care plans to be organised at a local level.

But doubts about the overall philosophical and political objectives as well as the practicalities of the organisation of the policy remain. Many writers (Finch and Groves, 1983; Dalley, 1988; Ungerson, 1987) have argued that the philosophical concept behind the policy was to replace the traditional gendered roles within the family and to focus upon the unpaid caring work of women as the main providers. Indeed it was explicitly stated in a government document in 1981 (Cmnd 8173, p. 3) that 'care in the community must increasingly mean care by the community' . The plight of informal carers, the majority of whom were women, was taken up by the National Association of Carers which published a report on the health and social problems experienced by carers (*Guardian*, 22 May 1992, p. 4). Politically, the suspicion was that the policy had been undertaken in order to lessen the cost of care for the social groups singled out for care in the community. As Mary Langan stated (1993) 'the central concern of the government is not to improve the quality of care but to reorganise community care in the interests of reducing overall social services expenditure'. Indeed, the government had always argued that a policy of community care was cheaper than institutional care. The Audit Commission in 1986 had estimated that elderly people could be cared for in their own homes at half the cost of a long-stay bed in a geriatric ward. But this is rejected by many who argue that high-quality community care delivered professionally and efficiently is not a cheaper option and that it only can be so if the work is done by unpaid or low-paid carers.

The plight of mentally ill people released from long-stay institutions into 'the community' was perhaps the most visible, and was the cause of much adverse publicity during 1993 and 1994. People with mental health problems were highly represented among the homeless and vagrants in most cities. There were also some much-publicised events concerning released patients, among them the Zito case where a man suffering from schizophrenia murdered a young man in a tube station and another where a person with a similar disorder climbed into the lions' den in London Zoo and was badly mauled. Events such as these have caused public concern and questioning over the policy of community care in respect of mentally ill patients, but in terms of numbers this is a minority group – it is elderly people who form the largest group in receipt of community care.

It is in the field of care of the elderly that the commercial or private sector has become dominant. The commercial provision of residential care rose significantly during the 1980s with the bulk of the fees being claimed from Social Security. Local authorities and not Social Security are now responsible for the fees in residential homes and there is growing evidence that families are being required to 'top up' payments for residential care. Often the responsibility for an older relative may cause tension and added worry for women with young families themselves.

The midwifery services which may not have been directly affected by the Community Care Act, may be given a more 'community-orientated approach' by some of the proposals of the *Changing Childbirth* report. This will be discussed in more detail in Chapter 8.

The concept of 'the community' is one which has become a part of recent social policy. The shift in emphasis from care by the State to care by the community has been the subject of much debate. Critics argue that this has meant a further burden to be placed upon women in families who make up the majority of unpaid care-givers. Women of course also make up the majority of professional care-givers in the community as community midwives, health visitors, district nurses and home care assistants. Chapter 7 focuses upon the way in which social policies have particular relevance to women's lives.

■ Questions and discussion points

- Poverty is a major cause of mortality and morbidity around childbirth. How could changes in social policy and benefit payments improve this situation?

- How would a midwife help a young single woman to trace her natural mother?
- How has the work of the Child Support Agency improved the health of mothers and their babies?
- Why do you think that the comments made in the House of Commons Health Committee Report (1992) about socio-economic factors in childbirth were not addressed by the DOH (1993) *Changing Childbirth* report?
- It has been argued that poverty could be reduced if the government were to provide subsidised child care. Discuss the advantages and disadvantages of such a scheme.
- What are the advantages and disadvantages of easier divorce?
- Suggest reasons for the poor take-up of some benefits.
- What is the rationale for care in the community?
- What are the principles of the Children Act?
- How can midwives assist women in taking up benefits to which they are entitled?
- Should mothers of babies born outside marriage be forced to give them up for adoption? Should the State support illegitimacy through benefits to unsupported mothers?

Key points

- In Britain, social policy is framed on a model of the family where gender roles have been institutionalised within legislation.
- The organisation and application of 'the male earner female dependent relationship', as defined by Beveridge in 1942, underpins many areas of social security, employment, childcare and taxation legislation.
- Social legislation in the 1960s and 1970s made divorce easier to obtain.
- Working women contribute to family income and this has had the effect of reducing poverty.
- In Social Security policies women's income is seen as 'extra' and therefore deductible from families' entitlement to benefit. This adds to the numbers caught in the so-called 'poverty trap'.
- The take-up of all means-tested benefits varies, except for Child Benefit where most eligible mothers claim.
- The Social Fund, set up in 1988, offered loans and 'start up' grants. Repayment is usually made by deductions from benefits.
- Families with disabled children can apply for grants from the Family Fund. As many as four in ten eligible families do not apply.
- In 1991 amidst controversy, dissent, hostility and public outcry the Child Support Agency was set up. It was subsequently modified.
- In 1991 there were approximately 75 000 children in local authority care in the UK. The Children Act gave rights to adopted children to seek birth information.

- The 1980s showed a determined shift of health care from hospitals to the 'community'.
- It has been argued that one of the effects of the NHS and Community Care Act 1990 was to place the burden of care of an increasingly elderly population as well as the sick and disabled on informal, unpaid, usually female, carers.
- Women, who may also be mothers, or expectant mothers now form the majority of unpaid carers. The traditional image of the male breadwinner providing for his wife and child is out of date.

Chapter 7

Women and social policy

As we saw in Chapter 6, British social policy has largely focused upon women as mothers rather than as workers or independent citizens. The relationship between the aims of social policies and the reality of women's lives is a complex one. Writers have pointed to the significance which social policies have for women's lives (Maclean and Groves, 1991; Williams, 1989). A broadly feminist perspective could be divided as to the way in which women should be identified by policies: for example, does a policy such as child benefit reinforce the gendered nature of child care or should it be protected as it represents the only benefit to which women are entitled as of universal right?

There are divisions within feminist thought on this type of question, and as Dale and Foster (1986) show, there is a whole spectrum of feminist analyses from that of the liberal to that of the radical feminists. Broadly speaking, a liberal orientation would be aimed at giving women *equality* with men on a formal basis (by outlawing sexual discrimination in employment for example) whereas a more radical perspective would argue for legislation to discriminate actively in favour of women, which would recognise the specific nature of women's lives (legislation on child-care provision) and without which women cannot possibly attain a measure of equality.

This chapter will concentrate on three main areas of social policy:

1. the pro-natalist policies which actively prescribed the mothering role for women;
2. policies which aimed to give a measure of formal equality;
3. policies which did not specifically target women but which had great significance for them.

As will be seen, it is difficult to categorise social policies in this way as all the policies to be discussed contain the implicit assumption that the role of women in the family is of dominating and overriding importance. All women are initially identified as potential, present or past wives and mothers. However, there are some policy areas which make this identification more explicit than others.

In looking at pro-natalist policies we shall examine the legislation on contraception, abortion, and recent measures on maternity benefits. The attempts to legislate for equality, both at work and in other areas of social life, will be illustrated by the equal opportunity and sexual discrimination policies and also those on the provision of child care which is closely related to the success of these. Finally, we give an analysis of the 'feminisation' of poverty and a questioning of the relevance of policies on housing and social security which have been a contributing factor. But before we look in depth at the content and structure of such policies, it is important to begin by addressing the central question of the place of women in the public world of the legal rights and duties of citizenship. Do women as a gender possess citizenship ?

■ Women and citizenship

What exactly does citizenship mean ? Historically, the concept emerged with the advent of the nation-state in the ferment of the French Revolution. There it had connotations of equality before the law and of a democratic system. But as Juliet Mitchell (1976) has pointed out, when this was transferred to the British context in the eighteenth century it lost any universal application which it may have previously suggested. In other words, when the 'Rights of *Man*' was published and the foundations of the practice of common law and justice were being laid down it was the rights of the 'Freeborn English*man*' which were to be protected. Citizenship then was based upon ideas of social worth and this meant ownership of property. The original concept of citizenship then was limited to male property owners. Very few women could own property in their own right, they did not inherit and on marriage they lost any claim to their own money. Women *were* property.

During the campaigns by the suffragettes for the vote, the opponents of female suffrage pointed to the fact than men were required to fight and possibly die for their country in time of war, whilst women were exempt from military service. Thus the right of citizenship was countered by the duty of a man to serve his country. How then could women attain the rights of citizenship? As we have seen in previous chapters it was as mothers that women gained a toehold on the notion of the rights of citizenship.

T.H.Marshall (1963) set out the three elements of citizenship in his famous thesis; these were:

• civil rights,
• political rights
• social rights.

As Marshall himself recognised, women as a gender lagged far behind men in the attainment of all of these elements.

The civil rights of the liberty of the person, freedom of speech, the right to own property, the right to conclude valid contracts and the right to work in a 'chosen trade' were historically prohibited to women. The *formal* equality of women before the law was and still remains, tempered by *informal* assumptions and prejudices which can mean that women are treated differently and sometimes more harshly than men (Kennedy, 1992).

The political rights of women were much more delayed than·those of men. The vote was 'given' to women aged 30 (men at 21) in 1918 and it was not until 1930 that women received the vote on the same basis as men. Even today, the number of women in Parliament is very low compared with men, as is female representation on Committees, Boards of Trusts and in Trade Unions.

The social rights of citizenship included the right to a basic standard of economic welfare and security, the right to share in one's social heritage and culture and access to institutions of education and social security. Although, as we shall see, great strides have been made by women in these areas, poverty still remains an essentially 'feminine' experience.

Ruth Lister (1991) has strongly argued that women have not attained a measure of equality of citizenship and are still regarded as a separate group for whom specific legislation is required. She argues that female dependency is built into the welfare system and that the idea of women as independent citizens is an ambiguous one. She points out that official literature often refers to 'individuals and their families' which clearly delegates women as on a par with children in their dependency. But as Lister argues, the concepts of independency, self-help and self-reliance formed the keystone of the political philosophy of the New Right administrations of the 1990s. This has meant contradictions for many women, the exhortations to be independent and not to rely on others has meant that in some ways women's lives have been disadvantaged by the lack of State provision of certain benefits, but in other ways women have gained a new sense of identity and assertiveness. Before looking at these complex issues, however, we turn to a review of the policies which could be said to have been overwhelmingly pro-natalist in assumption and practice.

■ Policies on contraception and abortion

For policy-makers of the nineteenth and early twentieth century, both contraception and abortion were seen as being two sides of the same practice and in reality, although shrouded in secrecy and taboo, both were widely practised. The desirability of promoting the limitation of families was fraught with contradictions and ideological problems. Since the end of the nineteenth century there had been growing public and political concern over what came to be called 'the population question' (Weeks,

1981). At a time when the birth-rate was decreasing, attention turned to the objective of producing a *quality* population. The new 'science' of eugenics gained many followers with the belief that a high-quality population could be produced by 'selective breeding'. This in effect meant that the connection between fertility and intelligence and social worth was believed to be irrefutable and the main problem for eugenicists was to promote breeding among one section of the population and to limit or prevent elements of the 'social problem group' from reproducing. So at the same time as policies on limiting the access of the majority of the population to contraception and abortion were applied, so there were proposals made for the compulsory sterilisation of the 'unfit'. These debates were very prominent in Britain throughout the period from the end of the nineteenth century to the Second World War.

However, both contraception and abortion were widely practised. It was obvious that the professional middle-classes practised some form of birth control by the end of the nineteenth century, and abortion (although illegal) was the most common form of contraception for the mass of the population.

Contraceptive devices had been available for many centuries but mostly only to men as a protection against venereal disease and for use only with prostitutes (MacLaren, 1978). By the end of the nineteenth century, advertisements for contraceptives began to appear in public but doctors were forbidden to give contraceptive advice to patients. Indeed the medical profession rejected any taint with such a controversial and shady subject and contraception remained a 'fringe' and disreputable area of health care. During the First World War condoms were issued to troops serving in France in an attempt to cut the enormous toll of venereal disease. This inevitably led to a wider dissemination of information amongst working-class people and was probably the origin of the description of condoms as 'French letters'.

During the 1920s, the number of groups set up to promote birth control among all social classes proliferated and clinics began to appear in many large towns. Respectable women's organisations such as the National Council of Women gave their support to birth control in 1929 and slowly it began to be a more accepted practice. The medical profession also began to give contraceptive advice, although the majority of doctors had received no formal education in contraception in their medical training.

In 1930 the Family Planning Association was formed, with the express purpose of giving information on the *spacing* of children within a marriage rather than the limitation of numbers. Even as late as the 1950s advice was only available to *married* or engaged women, and often they would be required to produce evidence of their status. The most used form of contraception available to women was the Dutch cap which required them to attend a clinic under the supervision of a doctor, be examined and receive 'training' in its use from a nurse. This effectively 'medicalised' female-based birth control and placed it within the respectable orbit of married family life.

The development of the contraceptive pill in the early 1960s revolutionised birth control practice. Although effectively giving women more autonomy it was firmly placed within the sphere of professional medical control as it became available on prescription only. The Brook Clinic opened in London in the 1960s and was the first to offer access to contraception to all women with no restrictions on age or marital status. This pattern of open access became the norm for medical practice too and most doctors would prescribe the pill to women on the same basis if they were clinically suitable. The prescribing of contraceptives for unmarried girls under the age of 16 without their parents' permission was challenged in 1984 by Mrs Victoria Gillick in an action taken against the Department of Health and Social Security. In a much-publicised action she gained a ruling from the High Court which required doctors to seek parental permission before prescribing the pill to under-aged girls. This was opposed by the BMA and was overturned on appeal to the House of Lords in 1985.

The Dutch cap had been the first birth control device for women and with the advent of the pill and the coil, contraception became primarily a female responsibility firmly controlled by the medical profession. This, of course, is in contrast to male contraceptives such as the condom which have always been openly available for purchase. In recent years, condoms have gained a measure of 'respectability' and have become even more widely available from slot machines, supermarkets and garages. This has been prompted by the AIDS campaigns and is more associated with protection from infection rather than control of conception which remains a female based and medically controlled practice. The female condom, though widely available has not been a runaway success; many women appear to dislike it as a form of contraception.

Abortion has been the subject of great controversy and policy legislation since the nineteenth century (Brookes, 1988). Some social historians (Mohr, 1984), argue that prior to the medical definition of abortion becoming prominent, it was not seen as morally or legally wrong. Brookes (1988) reveals that it was undoubtedly the main method of birth control practised *by women* during this time. Under the Abortion Act 1803, abortion was deemed illegal after 'quickening' – this rather vague term was taken to signify life. This meant that any terminations performed before this time were not really seen as a legal responsibility. The most popular methods of termination were the taking of various abortifacients such as: slippery elm, drugs like pennyroyal, the taking of diachylon (lead plaster) was said to be widespread in the Midlands, and gunpowder which was swallowed with margarine was also practised. The taking of hot baths, drinking gin, and as a 'last resort' the use of knitting needles and skewers were other methods. A distinction was made not only in the popular mind, but also in the legal sphere between taking pills and drugs to 'bring on a period' and the use of instruments. As with contraception, various pills and potions were advertised openly, women's magazines advertised 'cures for female irregularity' and Beecham's Pills were the most successful patented product. How widespread the practice of abortion by these methods was, is of course unknowable, but a study of women attending an out-patients' department in York in 1901 showed that eight out of ten mainly working-class women regularly took abortifacients. In 1823, the use of instruments to procure a termination was forbidden, but this was almost impossible to prove and the taking of drugs remained outside the law. The medical profession was gaining in power by the middle of the century and the passing of the Offences Against the Person Act of 1861 which set life imprisonment as the punishment for attempting to procure an abortion for both the woman and the practitioner, has been seen as the way in which the newly aspiring profession sought to exclude abortionists from its ranks. The use of instruments now became the basis for prosecution and although most 'professional abortionists' were men who operated among an affluent society clientèle, the amateur practising among a working-class clientèle was usually female and often, a midwife. Abortion then became a problem for the medical profession. Clinically, it could be said to be relatively safe but politically and professionally it was a subject of great controversy.

After the First World War, abortion rates appeared to be on the increase, probably because of the growth of unemployment and poverty and also the fact that a widow's pension would be withdrawn if she had a child. The increase in abortions probably contributed to the rise in maternal mortality rates during the 1930s. In 1934, it was calculated that the annual number of abortions was around 68 000 with only 33 convictions and 521 deaths. The investigation into fatalities revealed some startling facts: in one factory in Rotherham women paid into a weekly club to pay for an abortion. Because of the rise in mortality rates, the difficulties of prosecution and the opposition of some doctors to the law, opposition began to grow. In 1933, Judge McCardie publicly criticised the abortion laws and ruled that the woman did not have to give evidence in a prosecution or herself be prosecuted. The Abortion Law Reform Society was formed in 1935. In 1938, a well-known surgeon and opponent of the abortion law, Alec Bourne, voluntarily gave himself up for arrest after performing an abortion on a 15-year-old rape victim. The subsequent publicity led to a change in the law and in 1938 'therapeutic' abortions became legal. These were judged to be permissable if the life of the mother was in danger and/or there was evidence of mental handicap. The decision as to who could have a termination now lay firmly within the medical profession, but married women were more likely than others to get a termination.

In 1940, Stella Browne founded the Abortion Law Reform Association (ALRA) and argued for ' a woman's right to choose'. Agitation for a more liberal abortion system grew throughout the 1950s and 1960s, and in 1967, David Steel on behalf of the ALRA and supported by the BMA , the GMC, the Royal College of Nursing and Royal College of Midwives brought forward a private member's bill to allow abortion on mental health grounds. This bill which was passed and became law in 1967 allowed a termination to take place within 28 weeks if two doctors agreed that the mental health of the mother was at risk. In 1989, David Alton acting on behalf of the Society for the Protection of the Unborn Child (SPUC), brought forward a private members bill to reduce the time-limit to 20 weeks; this was defeated, but a new time limit of 22 weeks was agreed.

Abortion remains a controversial and highly politicised issue. As we saw in Chapter 4, the development of new technologies such as the scan have brought a new dimension to society's image of the fetus. This has fuelled much debate and even violence in the USA about the civil rights of the fetus as opposed to that of the mother. As Rachel Roth (1993) has argued, the two 'rights' can in fact be seen to be in opposition to each other. Generally speaking, those who focus upon the rights of the fetus do so from a right-wing perspective whilst the left focuses upon a woman's right. Opposition to abortion has been viewed as a backlash against feminism. The 'abortion question' has become one of central importance within the political agendas of both major parties in the USA but so far, has not taken on such a high profile within political debate in Britain.

Like birth control, abortion is a medically controlled practice with the GP as the 'gatekeeper' to both. Although the pro-natalist motivation behind policies which was evident in the early part of the century has disappeared and a high birth-rate is no longer seen as desirable, women have not gained complete 'mastery' of their own fertility. But although they remain subject to decisions taken by a male-dominated Parliament and by the medical profession, women have nevertheless gained immeasurably in autonomy and control over conception in the past thirty years, and as we have seen (Chapter 5) an increasing number of women are choosing to remain childless or perceive their working lives as being compatible with motherhood.

■ Maternity benefits

There are currently two kinds of maternity benefit available to working women. The first type, statutory maternity pay (SMP) is payable by the employer and the second type, maternity allowance (MA) is payable by Social Security. To qualify for SMP a woman must have been employed by the same employer for at least 26 weeks prior to and including the 15th week prior to the birth. She must also have been paying National Insurance contributions which means that her earnings must be at or above the lower earnings limit for the payment of NI contributions. The payment is at present (1995) 99 per cent of the average weekly earnings for the first six weeks only, if the woman has been employed on a full-time basis for the past two years or part-time for the past five years. After the initial six weeks a flat rate is paid for the following twelve weeks. To receive this payment women do not have to return to work after the birth although the employer must keep the post 'open' if the woman wishes to resume work. This policy effectively rewards those women who are in relatively well-paid and regular employment and who have a continuous employment record, although they will still be financially disadvantaged as the payment will not equal their previous salary. It seriously disadvantages women in low-paid, temporary part-time posts. These are posts commonly reserved for women. It can also be argued that those who have the greatest needs of state benefits – i.e. the poor – are least likely to receive them. Poor women are doubly disadvantaged when they become pregnant (see also Chapter 2).

Women who are self-employed or who do not have a continuous employment record may be entitled to the second type of benefit, the MA. This is a lower rate of payment and is dependent upon the woman having paid 26 weeks of NI contributions in the previous 66 weeks.

The payment of maternity benefits and the granting of statutory maternity leave has undoubtedly benefited a proportion of working women, but only those who have a relatively secure position in the employment structure. It has been argued that this advantage can be two-edged. Does the increase in employer's liability to pay maternity pay and give leave of absence make them wary of employing younger women especially in well-paid and full-time posts? The questioning of women applicants at interview as to their 'plans' for childbearing is against both the letter and the spirit of equal opportunity legislation, although as many women will testify, it is frequently done. There is also the fact that the gendered nature of 'parenting' is reinforced by the granting of *maternity* leave only and no recognition is given in Britain to *paternity* leave. The role of fatherhood is once again pushed to the periphery and in 1994, Britain firmly rejected EU legislation to implement a system of paternity leave such as those operating in other EU countries.

In British social policy the exclusion of men from leave for child care reinforces the traditional model of the male breadwinner. Children are seen as an individual responsibility rather than a social one which is shared by society as a whole. The payment of maternity benefit is obviously an example of a policy of 'special' treatment for women as they obviously have the responsibility for childbearing but social policies have also reinforced the role of women as child-rearers.

We move now to look at those policies which single out the needs of women as being of specific importance. These are policies (or lack of them) on child care and on equal opportunities and sex discrimination.

■ Child care

Men have never been required to take an active and designated part in child-rearing; popular ideologies and policies have firmly placed the 'hands-on' care of children with women. There is no place within the everyday life of our society for a man caring for small children. If we look at the provision of toilet facilities in shops, restaurants and other public places we find that all the baby-changing rooms are placed in female toilets. Children's clothes and goods are placed adjacent to those of women in large department stores with the men's departments usually on a separate floor. This arrangement with which we are all familiar and probably take for granted, is reflected in the public and private provision of child care.

Men are not usually employed in nurseries or playgroups and are often viewed with suspicion if they apply. In primary education, men are very much in a minority, although they are vastly overrepresented in head teacher posts. And yet the majority of paediatricians, child psychologists, professional child-rearing experts and those working in child protection have traditionally been men. But this is not due to a belief that men are 'natural' child-rearers, in fact the opposite, it is to a belief that women *normally* take care of children and it is only in specialised areas that the expertise and status of the male expert is deemed essential. The same position can be seen in another traditional female role, that of cooking. The majority of women for the majority of occasions are seen as the 'natural' providers of food but in specialist (and highly paid) areas, male expertise is required. These assumptions about the naturalness of gender attributes have fed into the response of British social policies towards the provision of publicly funded child care.

Both world wars led to an increase in the employment of women and to a corresponding increase in the provision of child care. During the 1914–18 War, the Treasury paid for up to 75 per cent of the costs of nursery provision for munitions workers and by 1917 there were 108 day nurseries provided in England and Wales. These gradually closed after the war. During the Second World War, the same pattern of provision was repeated. In 1940 there were 14 day nurseries and by 1943 there were 1345. The provision of child care accompanied by other provisions such as factory canteens, expanded school meals service, after-school activities, holiday homes schemes and paid shopping breaks were seen as essential if mothers were to be persuaded to work (Riley, 1984).

Despite increased demands for labour after the war, the provision of nurseries was withdrawn. Women were now required, as illustrated by the

Beveridge Report (1942), to be full-time wives and mothers at home.

During the 1950s there was a spread of psychological theories of 'maternal deprivation' (Bowlby, 1953) (see also Chapter 5) which accompanied a moral panic on so-called 'latchkey' children. So although there was a decrease in the numbers of married women and especially mothers working outside the home, those who continued to work were often beset by guilt and worry. One of the outcomes was to place child-minding mostly with the maternal grandmother and for women to take up predominantly part-time work.

The Plowden Report in 1967 gave strong support for the expansion of nursery education but gave priority to part-time education so as not to interfere with maternal bonding. Between 1975 and 1985 however, nursery education increased by 47 per cent and there is currently full- and part-time provision for 50 per cent of 3-year-olds and 90 per cent of 4-year-olds. But there are wide regional variations in nursery education and 'part-time' tends to be the dominant pattern.

In 1994, the Government announced its intention to increase provision for 3–5 year olds but this was not to be fully funded.

In 1995, the intention to issue vouchers (up to the value of £1000) for all 4-year-olds to receive some form of nursery education was announced. Critics argued that the majority of 4-year-olds receive nursery education any way and that it is the 3-year-olds who need more access to nursery education. Also great regional and local differences in availability of nurseries exist and some more affluent parents who currently purchase nursery education (at approximately £3000 per year) will be the only ones to benefit from such a system. There remains inadequate funding of a universal and national system of nursery education for all and there are no plans to extend state nursery education to children under 4-years of age.

Public nurseries experienced a changing role after 1968. After that date, priority was given to children of single parents or other socially disadvantaged groups. Children with special needs and those defined as 'at risk' have increasingly dominated the places. By 1983, 75 per cent of children in public day nurseries had been referred by health visitors or social services. Very often these nurseries have been redesignated as Family Centres. Most parents of children placed there are not at work and the therapy often requires their attendance and so they are not nursery provision for working mothers.

Playgroups which evolved in the 1960s are extremely widespread and greatly utilised throughout Britain. They are, however criticised by some (Finch, 1984) as having prevented properly funded nursery education from being implemented as they represent ideas of self-help and individual action. They are little used by mothers who work full-time as the majority do not operate during suitable hours. Also many expect mothers (rarely fathers) to contribute on a rota basis. Most are non-profit-making and are run by parents or church groups; some are commercially run but only a very small proportion are operated by social services. Children attend on an average 2–3 times a week for about 2–4 hours at a time. They are in term-time only with little provision for holidays and there are more in rural and suburban areas than in the inner cities. There are also great regional variations in both standards and provision. Playgroups were at first to be excluded from the provision for pre-school child vouchers, but new legislation in 1995 allowed for their inclusion.

Registered *childminders* represent an important sector of the child-care provision. In 1986 it became mandatory for local authorities to register and also to inspect the properties and facilities offered by childminders. In 1986 there were approximately 66 000 registered childminders in England and Wales. Most of these were women aged under 40 with children of their own. No qualification or training is necessary and there is no fixed rate of pay, which usually reflects the 'going rate' for the area. Some local authorities sponsor childminders or give grants.

However, the vast majority of childminding remains informal with the husband/partner supplying care if the mother works part-time or shifts and with the maternal grandmother/grandparents if working full-time. (see Table 7.1).

A few firms or establishments offer *workplace nurseries* and a recent development has been *child-care vouchers*. But both these facilities are generally only offered to highly trained staff whose skills are in great demand. Tax changes in 1988 meant that nursery provision was judged as a taxable benefit for all employees earning over £8 500 per year and employer subsidies were withdrawn. In 1994, the Government brought in a new *child care allowance* which was intended to aid women in getting back to work and off benefits. It is only payable to those receiving family credit, housing benefit and supplementary benefit and only to pay for a registered childminder or nursery.

Table 7.1 Childcare arrangements for women employees with youngest child under 5, 1990, per cent

Workplace nursery	–
Day nursery	17
Mother works from home	5
Children look after themselves until mother gets home	–
Mother works only while children at school	8
Mother's help/nanny	7
Childminder	17
Friend/neighbour	1
Relative	64*

* Percentages sum to 119 because more than one form of care could be used.

Sources: Adapted from Witherspoon and Prior (1991), p. 139; S. Holterman and R. Clarke, *Parents' Employment Rights and Childcare* (EOC, 1992).

The pattern of child-care provision in Britain is very fragmented and, many would argue, totally inadequate. Nursery provision in Britain lags far behind that of most other EU countries and supporters of equal opportunities maintain that lack of public child care is the single biggest cause of low-paid part-time employment of women and of the ensuing poverty trap.

■ Equal opportunities and sex discrimination

During the 1970s, legislation was passed which sought to restrict both discrimination on the grounds of sex and also the gap between men's and women's earnings: these were the *Equal Pay Act*, 1970 (implemented 1975) and the *Sex Discrimination Act*, 1975. *The Equal Opportunities Commission* (EOC) was also set up in 1975 to monitor sex discrimination in many areas including education, training and employment. The EOC acts on behalf of women (and men) who feel that they have been unjustly discriminated against because of their sex. It also sponsors research into areas of discriminatory practice and produces many reports on topics as diverse as the plight of informal carers to the lack of women in science and technology. Similar equal opportunities policies had been put into practice a decade before in the USA and by the 1970s all EC countries followed suit, some countries such as Sweden were comparatively advanced in their attitudes and practices.

The Equal Pay Act was introduced at a time when the gap between the relative hourly pay of female and male workers was actually closing (from around 60 per cent to 70 per cent between the early and the late 1970s). The Act made it illegal for employers to pay women less than men doing the same or a 'broadly similar' job. This provision limited the scope of the Act to make actual inroads into wage disparity. The British labour market has historically been based upon a high degree of segregation, that is most jobs are male- or female-dominated (Gluckman, 1990; Walby, 1986). This meant that the necessity to prove that she was doing a job which was 'like work' was a great deterrent to many women. Also the delay of five years between the Act (1970) and its actual implementation meant that many employers further regraded and redefined jobs done by different workers in order to eradicate possible similarities. Not surprisingly the number of claims made by women dropped from 1 742 in 1975 to only 39 in 1982.

There is an argument that the rise in women's pay during the 1970s was because of legislation affecting low-paid workers as a whole and the restrictions on free collective bargaining which benefited white male skilled workers and had very little to do with the Equal Pay Act. After much lobbying, the Act was amended in 1983 to come in line with EC directives. *The Equal Pay Amendment Act* 1983 altered the wording to 'equal pay for work of equal value' but again this has so far had little real effect as the onus remains upon the worker to illustrate this fact. Despite the increased activity of women in the labour market the overall differential between men's and women's earnings remains at around 75 per cent.

The Sex Discrimination Act 1975 made it illegal to deny entry to educational establishments or careers to women. This made it illegal for medical schools to operate the quota system which had been in operation and for universities to bar women from science and engineering courses. Schools also had to offer a 'non-sexist' curriculum and to open subjects such as domestic science and woodwork to both boys and girls. Many commentators viewed the education system as the root cause of sex discrimination in all aspects of society (Stanworth, 1983; Deem, 1978). Despite some changes after 1975, mixed schools, it is argued, continue to operate a hidden curriculum of sex discrimination, which effectively discourages girls from entering 'male' subjects like maths and sciences and equal access to sports facilities. Recently, research by the DES has shown that girls benefit from single-sex education and that the moves towards mixed schools after the 1970s actually further advantaged boys.

So we can see that despite formal legislation on equal pay and anti-discrimination, the relative disadvantage experienced by women remains. Have equal opportunity policies failed ?

A wide-ranging survey of equal opportunities legislation in Europe and America (Sloane and Jain, 1989) concluded that in most cases legislation followed but did not initiate improvements in women's pay and opportunities. Nevertheless, as Dex and Shaw (1986) point out, legislation takes many years for changes following to be observable. As Dale and Foster (1986) argue, even 'small changes' in services will affect large numbers of women. Policies of formal equality are essential if only as a 'security net' or a base from which individual women can make gains for themselves and others.

Today, the cases involving sex discrimination tend to centre on accusations of sexual harassment and the rights of pregnant women and mothers. Many institutions now have policies regarding the reporting of sexual harassment and there have been some much-publicised cases.

The EU has been responsible for the imposition of compensation for sex discrimination suffered by British women which has had to be enforced by the British government. The most recent was the case of compensation for unlawful dismissal from the armed forces on the grounds of pregnancy. The highest award (£172 912) was that given to Mrs Nicola Cannock in 1994 by the RAF in lieu of her dismissal ten years previously. There is therefore some evidence to show that anti-discriminatory legislation will strengthen with Britain's inner membership of the EU.

In the 1990s, there were great changes in the labour market in Britain which mirrored the social changes. As women's employment, mostly in low paid and part-time jobs, grew apace, so men's employment in the full-time skilled manual sector, fell. Women's employment was characterised by two popular expressions; the 'glass ceiling' and the 'stone floor'. The 'glass ceiling' was said to affect relatively well-paid women in the professions and in public and private sector management who found it almost impossible to be promoted above a middle level. The 'stone floor' was the position of the majority of working-class women who were concentrated either in low-paid jobs or who existed on state benefits. What was the effect of policies on women who existed on the margins of poverty ?

■ Women and benefits

The 'invisibility' of women in social policies is best illustrated by looking at the composition of groups living in poverty. Over seventy years ago the welfare campaigner, Eleanor Rathbone, stated that 'children are the main cause of women's poverty', and this still remains largely the case. Despite all the welfare reforms and the introduction of policies on social security, unemployment pay, sick pay and pensions since 1945, women have increasingly made up the larger part of those living in poverty. In the late 1980s, Heather Joshi reported that a woman who has two children will forego average earnings of £122 000 over her lifetime (Joshi, 1987). This is the price of female dependency which still remains largely invisible.

Unlike the Beveridge Plan which, despite its failings, did address the position of women as something distinct, recent measures have tended to ignore the specificity of women's lives altogether. Figures on the sex differences in social security claims are very difficult to obtain. Millar and Glendinning (1987) argue that data on poverty has always concentrated on household incomes or families and have therefore marginalised the position of women as the main sufferers from poverty and its subsequent effects on health and well-being. Women as a group are most vulnerable to poverty when they are mothers, especially single and unsupported, and also in old age, but they are also more likely to be in individual poverty within a household or family which itself is above the official poverty line (Pahl, 1989).

Wynn (1995) points out that one baby in three is still born into a family defined as poor because they depend in whole or part on welfare benefits or have earnings less than half the average wage. She argues that in such families, the budget for food is squeezed to meet other costs such as warmth, rent and debts. She points out that the Beveridge report sought to rid the country of want and squalor but its policies have failed. She says: '40 per cent of babies are born to mothers under 25 years of age, 11 per cent to mothers under 20. From the point of view of preventative medicine, it is unbelievable that these mothers get lower levels of income support than those over 25!' (Wynn, 1995, p. 37). Yet the social security system is still very much dominated by women as recipients despite the fact that it was initially based upon men's working patterns and the ideal of the stable nuclear family.

As Table 7.2 demonstrates, women are the largest claimants of benefits.

In addition to these benefits, it is estimated that a further social security benefit of some type is paid to nearly 4 million married men to meet the needs of their wives (Essam and Berthoud, 1991). Within low-income families it is nearly always the woman who has the task of budgeting and managing the finances.

Since 1979, following an EC directive, women and men have been given 'equal treatment' in social security matters. But as Hilary Land (1986) has argued equal treatment does not necessarily mean 'equal outcomes'. Women's and men's lives are distinctly different in terms of employment patterns and domestic responsibilities and this often means that a 'gender-blindness' in the benefit system actually further disadvantages many women.

The system remains based upon men's employment patterns and this means that women who are more likely to be in low-waged and part-time jobs will not gain parity in a contributory system based upon uninterrupted working lives and full contributions. Women who may work full-time but on an irregular basis may in fact pay 'wasted' contributions

Table 7.2 Social security claimants, by sex, Great Britain, 1990, per cent

Benefit	Women	Men
Income Support	57	43
Family Credit	99	1
Severe Disablement Allowance	60	40
Mobility Allowance	48	52
Invalid Care Allowance	82	18
One-Parent Benefit	91	9
Child Benfit	98	2
Attendance Allowance	63	37
Reduced Earnings Allowance	17	83
Widows Benefit	100	Nil
Unemployment Benefit	32	68
Sickness Benefit	26	74
Retirement Pension	65	35
Maternity Benefit	100	Nil
Invalidity Benefit	24	76
Industry Injury Disablement Benefit	11	89
Industrial Death Benefit	100	Nil

Source: Adapted from House of Commons, *Hansard* (1990), quoted in Lister (1992).

for which they can receive no benefits (Luckhaus and Dickens, 1991). In 1992, it was estimated that over 2 million working women were excluded from the contributory system altogether because they were earning below the limit (Lister, 1992). There remains of course a hidden army of home-workers about whom very little is known, who may work exceedingly long hours for very little pay and who are entitled to no benefits at all.

In 1986, the Fowler Review of the social security system was aimed at targeting resources at those most in need, the 'individualisation' of benefits and the cutting of public expenditure by encouraging the incentive to work. But once again as with the Beveridge Report forty years earlier, the specific circumstances of women's lives were not really addressed.

Unemployment benefit was altered in 1988 to base entitlement on previous work records. This had the effect of disadvantaging those with a short or disrupted record, the majority of whom are women. This resulted in a shortfall of money for claimants and in 1990 it was estimated that 50 per cent of female claimants failed to qualify, on the grounds of insufficient contributions (Lister, 1992). As commentators have noted (Land, 1986) the rules stipulating that a claimant must be 'available for work' meant that a person with child-care responsibilities had to show that child care was available immediately should a job be offered. If a woman argued that lack of settled care was a 'good cause' for her refusal of a job she could be deemed as unavailable for work (Bryson and Jacobs, 1992). The unemployment figures for women are usually accepted to be vastly underrated as many women who are either married or cohabiting do not bother to register because they would gain no benefit. Most women search for work on an informal basis, relying on word of mouth and recommendations of friends. This does not easily sit with the 'actively seeking work' clause of the 1989 Act.

Women are increasingly dependent upon means-tested benefits both as claimants and as managers of benefit money within a household. Since the 'equal treatment' clause was adopted in 1983, women have been able to claim supplementary benefit/income support on behalf of couples. In 1990, one in every twenty claims by a couple were made by the woman, although this proportion is low, it was one in 2000 in 1983 (Lister, 1992). One of the reasons for this low figure may be the need for the compliance of the husband which is required in order to make the claim. Research by Corden and Craig (1991) suggests that there are gender differences in the claiming of family credit with men being far more reluctant to claim than partners. The payment of family credit is also made through the main wage packet and so will be paid directly in most cases to the man. Women's hidden poverty could therefore continue even though this was not the intention of the original policy.

But the reduction in the number of hours which constitute full-time work, from 24 hours to 16 hours in 1992 will, it is estimated, have the effect of increasing the number of families in low-paid jobs who are entitled to family credit. But this will once again be determined by the agreement of male partners to reveal their earnings and to redistribute the extra income to the wife.

A life-experience of dependency, unpaid caring, low or infrequent economic activity has rendered many women especially vulnerable to poverty in old age. Current government changes in retirement and pension provision have largely ignored the specificity of women's lives. Low-waged and part-time work has been largely excluded from occupational pension schemes and the payment of a widow's pension scarcely recompenses for the loss of a man's wage or pension. On divorce, women also lost any access to their ex-husband's pension which was especially hard on women who divorced in late middle-age after a lifetime of unpaid work in the home. This is currently (1995) in the process of being altered by legislation which will give divorced wives a proportion of a husband's pension after a long period of marriage. Although increasingly women are making provision for their own pensions, the real benefit will only accrue to those in full-time and relatively well-paid careers. By the end of the century, the retirement ages for men and women will be equalised at 65 but this could further disadvantage low-paid women who will have to work for a further 5 years before receiving the state pension. Even when they receive a state pension at the current age of 60, women who receive invalidity benefit are disadvantaged. This benefit is higher than the state pension rate and women are forced to go on the lower rate five years earlier than men whose state pension is paid at the age of 65. This was recently (1995) unsuccessfully challenged in the EU court by a woman in this position.

Although there have been moves within the social security system to cut dependency and to encourage work, the low wages which most women can attain plus the lack of publicly funded child care mean that work is not always the rational economic option for many.

But this does not necessarily mean that work is not wanted or preferred by women themselves. (see Table 7.3). Meanwhile, the income for a single mother who is reliant on benefits are seen in Table 7.4.

The responsibility for managing low incomes falls disproportionately upon women. Recent research has shown (Craig and Glendinning, 1990, Cohen *et al.*, 1992) that women sacrifice their own well-being and needs for children and for the household as a whole. This everyday responsibility adds to the stress and sheer debilitating experience of managing poverty which is left mostly to women. As Craig and Glendinning state;

> Without exception women in the families carried the main burden of poverty. It was women family members who managed the budget, the women who went without when things were really tight and women who had to explain to children why they could not have the same Christmas

Table 7.3 Employment rates of lone mothers, actual and preferred, Great Britain, 1991, per cent

	Preferred employment rates			Actual employment rates		
	0–4*	5–9	10–15	0–4	5–9	10–15
All	40	61	73	21	47	65
Part-time	17	28	29	13	25	19
Full-time	23	33	44	9	22	46

* Age of youngest child.

Source: Adapted from J. Bradshaw and J. Millar, *Lone Parents in the UK* (HMSO, 1991).

presents as others. All too often it was also women who bore the brunt of family rows and tensions arising out of financial worries. (Craig and Glendinning, 1990, 30)

The housing of low-income families has also in recent years become more the responsibility of women.

■ Housing and homelessness

The sayings 'a woman's place is in the home' and 'an English*man*'s home is his castle' reflect accurately the place of women in housing policies. Allocation of rented public housing and ownership of private housing have both been placed firmly within the 'male breadwinner model'.

In the realm of public housing, for the greatest part of this century, council houses were allocated to married couples with children and as Marion Roberts (1991) has recorded, most inter-war and post-war estates were built in the suburbs where employment for women, unlike the urban areas, was virtually unobtainable. Housing allocation was based upon the patriarchal ideal that it was men who provided the wages to pay the rent and were therefore the sole or chief-named tenant. Women provided the

Table 7.4 Total weekly income, single mother and one child, from Income Support and Child Benefit*, Great Britain, 1995

	£
18 years and over at home or alone	73.60
16–18 years living alone	64.40
16 and 17 years living at home	56.05

* The figures do not include housing benefit.

Source: Adapted from *Social Policy Research*, 72 (1995).

'respectability' necessary, it was common practice for housing officers to select prospective tenants on the basis of housekeeping standards of cleanliness and good management.

Housing policies were firmly predicated upon a construction of the 'ideal' family life with strictly segregated gender roles – the male bread-winner in a steady job, who would spend free time in the garden or on house maintenance whilst the female carer's sphere of operation was indoors and preferably in the kitchen. Marion Roberts illustrates how the design of houses, and especially kitchens, in the 1950s were based upon this ideal type.

During the 1950s and 1960s, the growth of New Towns and vast housing estates coincided with the post-war baby 'bulge'. Many young couples from large urban areas were allocated houses in these new towns for the purpose of building a community. Harlow New Town in Essex, for example, became known as 'Pram Town' because Saturday afternoons would see a pram jam in the high street (Attfield, 1989). The emphasis in both pre- and post-war building was on houses for families rather than flats for single people or childless couples. This was a pro-natalist policy because, as Charles Mumford, the American city architect argued, family life should be given a priority in town planning and women discouraged from seeking employment outside the home. He advised:

> the first consideration of town planning must be to provide an urban environment and an urban mode of life which will not be hostile to biological survival: rather to create one in which processes of life and growth will be so normal to that life, so visible, that by sympathetic magic it will encourage women of child-bearing age the impulse to bear and rear children, as an essential attribute of their humanness, quite as interesting in all its possibilities as the most glamorous success in an office or factory. (Mumford, 1945)

The status of council housing throughout the 1950s and 1960s remained relatively high. It was mainly the respectable working-class family who inhabited estates and they were almost totally, white, with a man as head of household and employed. There were great social differences between estates which were well-known to most localities. Allocation to a 'good' estate was often seen as a badge of respectability to be distinguished from allocation to a 'slum clearance' estate which may have contained some 'rough' families (Roberts, 1991).

The desire by local authorities to impose a middle-class standard of living upon the tenants resulted in bans on hanging out washing in some areas. It was felt that this would lower the tone and it was seen as a part of a working-class lifestyle which was to be discouraged. How the mothers of small children managed to cope with the washing and drying is not recorded. One significant outcome however of such policies was the installation of drying cabinets inside flats which produced condensation and damp and were later designated as a cause of childhood chest complaints (Blackburn, 1991).

The social changes which occurred throughout the 1980s had a dramatic effect on housing allocation and on the social composition of housing estates and were especially significant for women. The 1980 Housing Act, the 'right to buy' legislation, encouraged council tenants to purchase their houses at very attractive rates. This was a central plank of the first Thatcher administration's electoral manifesto and was extremely popular with the electorate. But as later research has shown (Forrest and Murie, 1988), this popular move had very far-reaching and in some ways catastrophic consequences.

The houses purchased tended to be mainly of the 'best' stock – that is, those houses built to very high standards in the 1950s and 1960s leaving local authorities with the lower quality houses on increasingly rundown estates. The people who bought these houses were often the original tenants who were now middle-aged, with no dependent children left at home and who were still in relatively well-paid and secure employment. Overwhelmingly they were married couples with the husband taking out the mortgage in either his name or jointly. But of most significance for the future prospects of housing allocation, very little new house building was undertaken by rate-capped local authorities except for 'special needs' groups such as sheltered housing for the elderly or disabled.

At the same time, as we have seen, the divorce rate was rising, as was the rate of single motherhood and, of course, unemployment. All these factors came together in a social cocktail which had crucial effects on the composition and status of council housing estates. From being housing for the respectable working-class family from the 1930s to the 1960s, council housing in the 1980s and 1990s has become 'marginalised' and the site of the polarisation of social divisions.

One of the greatest changes has been the feminisation and impoverishment of local authority housing. As Table 7.5 shows, the increase in numbers of people in receipt of supplementary benefit in local authority housing grew dramatically between the 1970s and 1980s. Housing tenure became one of the biggest divisions between one parent and two parent families in the 1980s (see Figure 7.1).

By 1990 it was calculated that seven out of ten lone mothers lived in rented accommodation (Family Policy Studies Centre, 1990). Single mothers are far more likely to be allocated a flat than a house and these are likely to be on 'hard to let' estates. This has led to the ghettoisation of many single mothers on certain estates with all the attendant problems of safety, vandalism and lack of amenities this implies. This situation was prominently reported in the media in 1993 when the then Welsh Secretary, John Redwood, made an attack on such an estate in Cardiff.

Table 7.5 Supplementary Benefit recipients, by tenure, Great Britain, 1972 and 1984

Tenure	All recipients	Supplementary pensioners	Unemployed	Sick and disabled	Single parent families
1972					
Number (000)	2 482	1 796	269	183	164
	%	%	%	%	%
Owner-occupiers	17	18	14	14	7
LA tenants	55	53	53	60	63
Tenants of private landlords	29	29	33	26	30
1984					
Number (000)	3 389	1 550	1 069	151	425
	%	%	%	%	%
Owner-occupiers	21	22	22	22	14
LA tenants	61	61	55	65	75
Tenants of private landlords	17	16	23	13	12

Source: Forrest and Murie (1988). Reproduced by permission.

Black single mothers are also more likely to be allocated a flat in a high-rise block which is far above ground level.

Ironically, older women now widowed or caring for an elderly husband, who perhaps moved on to some estates in the 1950s as young mothers, now find themselves in the same situation, occupying a house in a now rundown estate and subject to harassment and fear.

Divorce generally disadvantages women in the housing market much more than it does men. As a rule because of their lower earning capacity most women cannot afford to pay a mortgage after divorce, and this lack of financial power is more acute for older women. If the family house remains with the wife until the youngest child is of school-leaving age, as some settlements have allowed, this often means that a woman in her fifties could find herself in danger of homelessness. Dependence on another male breadwinner by remarrying may be the only way for some women to remain in owner-occupation. Many divorced wives stay on in the original home with the mortgage being paid by the social services rather than herself, this has been the case with many 'clean-break' divorce settlements and is one of the causes of the rising social security costs. In this case, dependency of the woman remains a fact of her situation.

Until recently, many building societies were very reluctant to give mortgages to single women or even to include a wife's earnings in the mortgage allowance. By the late 1980s, however, these restrictions had

Figure 7.1 Home ownership, by household type, Great Britain, 1984 and 1991

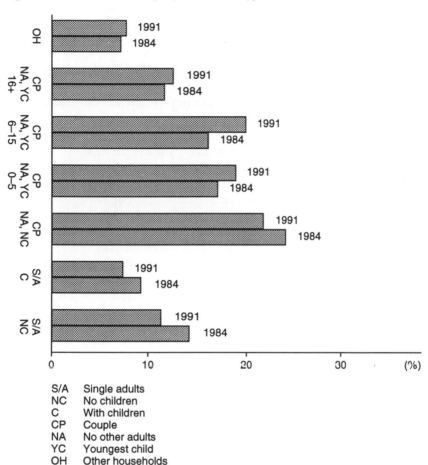

S/A	Single adults
NC	No children
C	With children
CP	Couple
NA	No other adults
YC	Youngest child
OH	Other households

Sources: Adapted from Joseph Rowntree Foundation, *Housing Research*, 134 (December 1994);
T. Hogarth and P. Elias, *Unemployment and Housing Tenure* (Institute of Employment Research, 1994).

largely disappeared and there is now some evidence that young single women under 30 outnumber young men as single owner-occupiers. This applies largely to childless and relatively well-paid women, so is it children which render women vulnerable to substandard housing and even homelessness?

Watson and Austerberry (1986), argue strongly that 'all women are potentially homeless' and by this they mean that women are likely to be 'sharing' a home with a male breadwinner especially if they have dependent children. This makes them more vulnerable to homelessness especially in cases of domestic violence and marriage break-up. Even if rehoused by local authorities following such a situation, women frequently occupy housing of a lower standard than that which they shared with a male partner. Women are often therefore rendered invisible in figures on homelessness as they may be occupying temporary accommodation (Greve, 1991).

There is far less provision for homeless vagrant women than for men. Homeless women are far less likely than men to apply for hostel accommodation. Greve reports that most hostels are alienating and even threatening to women as they were always intended as a provision for men only. Historically, homelessness among women was regarded as tantamount to prostitution (Watson and Austerberry, 1986). Many employers would offer 'live-in' accommodation to female servants, hotel workers or shop assistants. This also meant that they then paid correspondingly low wages and exercised complete control over their leisure and social life. This pattern was repeated in nurses' residential homes and in some universities and teacher training colleges until fairly recently. The institution such as a hospital could then exercise control and also extract long working hours from women – conditions which would have been totally unacceptable to male employees.

Most homeless people are young and during the 1980s and 1990s homelessness grew fastest among young people between the ages of 16 and 18. London is often the focus for studies on homelessness but in fact 78 per cent of households accepted as homeless in 1990 were living in other areas.

Despite women's economic disadvantage in the housing market, young men are in the majority of the 'roofless' population living rough on the streets. The majority have previously been in care and have mental health problems, young women however, are not (at present) so likely to be 'roofless', as friends and relatives are more inclined to offer temporary shelter to them. Young women are more likely to leave a family home than are young men, reasons include a breakdown in family relationships, sexual abuse and the incidence of pregnancy. Most young homeless women have a dependent child and this has given rise to a myth, much heard, that young women 'get themselves pregnant' in order to gain access to housing. Research however (Ermisch, 1990), has shown that about 75 per cent of single mothers were previously married and these form the bulk of single parents applying for accommodation.

Under the Housing (Homeless Persons) Act 1977, there is a statutory obligation upon local authorities to house homeless persons in their area. Among the categories of need priority was given to those with 'responsibility for dependent children' and this in an oblique way can 'advantage' women as they are more likely to have this responsibility. Single people would only be judged in need if they were 'vulnerable as a result of old age, mental illness or physical disability'. This left the definition of 'vulnerability' very narrow indeed and disqualified many who were victims of abuse at home.

In 1994, after a rousing speech at a Conservative Party Conference attacking single mothers who 'jumped the housing queue', new legislation on priority need was passed. Priority is now given to couples with responsibility for dependent children. Thus once again the primacy of the male breadwinner model (even if he is actually low paid or unemployed) is reasserted.

During the 1980s and early 1990s there was a great increase in the number of families (mostly of single parents) housed by local authorities. But the trend now is for short-term leasing arrangements such as in private-sector houses and mobile homes rather than in hostels or costly bed and breakfast accommodation. (see Table 7.6).

In 1990, in London alone, a population the size of Norwich was housed in some form of temporary accommodation.

Since the 1980s there has been a great increase in owner-occupation and a corresponding decrease in public or private renting. In 1994, over 65 per cent of housing in Britain was owner-occupied. Housing Associations have become an important agency in housing provision and have been instrumental in providing accommodation for many low-income groups. But rents can be high and this has had an effect on the cost of housing benefit. Repossessions of mortgaged homes also grew throughout the late 1980s and the experience of many families is that they are now on negative equity, owing more in mortgage repayments than the house is currently worth. But it is the new role of council housing as residual housing for the marginalised poor including single mothers which has been one of the most remarkable developments since 1980.

As we have seen from this overview, women occupy a contradictory role in social policies. They have either been the object of policies or have been the recipients of uncalculated effects of policies which have not allowed for the circumstances of women's domestic and working lives. The position of women has changed almost out of recognition since the foundation of the welfare state in 1945 but many anomalies still remain. Changes in the employment and family structures have meant that social policies have often been designed for a situation which no longer exists. The decline of the 'male breadwinner' looks to be permanent and this is possibly the single most important factor for change in policies on employment, family support, equal opportunities, child care and security in old age. It must be borne in mind that the decline in the male breadwinner has not been replaced by the female breadwinner. Most women work in lower paid and less secure jobs than men and unemployed men are more likely to have an unemployed partner. In a dual earner household, women's wages represent a higher proportion of a household income than they did previously, but they still do not match those of employed men.

The debate in social policy therefore centres around the way in which women should be defined. Should policies attempt to 'equalise' the economic and social status of men and women ?

Table 7.6 Households living in temporary accommodation, England, 1982–92, end-year data*

Year	Hostels (000)	Bed and breakfast (000)	Short-life leasing (000)	Total (000)
1982	3.5	1.6	4.2	9.3
1983	3.4	2.7	3.7	9.8
1984	4.0	3.7	4.6	12.3
1985	4.7	5.4	5.8	15.9
1986	5.2	9.0	7.2	20.8
1987	10.4	10.4	9.2	24.8
1988	6.2	11.0	12.9	30.1
1989	8.0	11.5	18.4	37.9
1990	9.0	11.1	25.1	45.3
1991	10.0	12.2	37.8	59.9
1992	10.7	7.7	44.5	62.9

* Includes households awaiting outcome of homeless enquiries.

Source: Adapted from *Social Trends*, 24 (1994).

If this approach is adopted then a programme of 'positive' discrimination will be essential in order to bring women up to parity with men. This will mean discriminating in favour of women in employment and education. This has been implemented to some degree in the US with much opposition. In Britain, the imposition by the New Labour Party of 'women only' short lists for vacant candidatures has aroused great controversy and antagonism from both male and female members.

The other alternative for policy-makers is to recognise that women have different life and working patterns and seek to address the 'special' nature of their lives via woman-friendly measures affecting child-care and benefits. But does this approach merely reinforce and reproduce the position of women as marginalised dependents? This debate is likely to be at the centre of the larger debate on the future of the welfare services in the next decade.

■ **Mothers in employment**

The House of Commons Employment Committee published its report 'Mothers in Employment' in March 1995. It received advice from many sources but one of the most important was the advice offered by the Maternity Alliance. In their publication 'Maternity Action' they set out the key recommendations of the report based to a large extent on the evidence supplied by them. The key points and recommendations are as follows:

1. The provision of maternity pay is fundamental to enabling women with dependent children to work. Some of the poorest women, with children, who need to be included in the benefit system are excluded. The recommendation is that the Government extends rights proportionately to women below the National Insurance threshold.
2. That the Government should overhaul and simplify the system of maternity pay, to make it accessible and understandable to employers and employees alike.
3. A single Government department should co-ordinate all issues relating to pregnancy and maternity provision.
4. Existing maternity pay and leave arrangements can have a serious effect on health of mothers and babies. All mothers should be entitled to 18 weeks leave.
5. The requirement placed on employers to reimburse the costs of maternity pay acts as a disincentive to recruit female employees of child bearing age and should be phased out.
6. There should be five days family leave and five days, paternity leave.

The Maternity Alliance and women of childbearing age everywhere await the government's response!

Case Study

Louise is pregnant for the second time. Her first child, now aged 18 months, was born with cystic fibrosis. She is separated from her husband, Bill, who as a police officer is being actively pursued by the Child Support Agency even though he pays her a regular sum in maintenance. Louise gave up her job as a clerk, which she had held for six months, when she became pregnant and when her first child's health deteriorated further. Louise is claiming benefits and has recently made an application to the social fund for a grant for maternity clothes.

At the GP surgery she is very tired, distressed and in need of some practical support. The midwife arranges for her to meet the practice social worker and asks the community nurse to make an assessment of her needs in relation to her first child.

She plans to divorce her husband and is seeking the advice of a solicitor in relation to custody of her daughter and unborn child.

■ Questions

- Is there anything else that the midwife can do to help Louise?
- Why is Louise not entitled to Maternity Pay?
- Who benefits most from Maternity Pay provision?
- In what circumstances are payments made from the social fund?

- Are there any charities, other organisations or self-help groups that might be able to help Louise?
- How does poverty effect pregnancy outcome?

■ Other questions and discussion points

- Social policies define women primarily as carers rather than earners. List the ways in which pregnant women are disadvantaged by this definition.
- Citizenship included civil, political and social rights. How are child-bearing women disadvantaged by their unequal social rights?
- Are women's political rights compromised by the small numbers of women in parliament?
- How have current maternity benefit policies disadvantaged some child bearing women?
- Discuss the arguments for and against paid paternity leave?
- How would a system of centrally funded nursery education for the under 3s benefit women?
- Has the equal pay and opportunities legislation worked in women's favour?
- Poverty is a major cause of perinatal mortality and morbidity. Why are single mothers especially vulnerable?
- What advice can a midwife offer to a young, pregnant, single woman on benefits?
- Suggest reasons why some single women choose to become pregnant.

Key points

- Social policy can be divided into three main areas.
  (i)   Pro natalist policies which actively define and prescribe the mothering role;
  (ii) Policies which aim to give some sort of equality;
  (iii) Policies not targeted at women but highly significant for them.
- In most, if not all, social policies is the implicit assumption that the role of women in the family is the most important.
- Women do not share equal rights of citizenship with men.
- Control of female fertility through contraception remains firmly in the hands of the medical profession.
- Abortion is medically controlled with access via GPs.
- Policies on maternity benefit currently favour women in well-paid, regular, secure, continuous employment.
- Maternity benefits and statutory maternity leave arrangements may encourage employers to take on older women or men rather than risk paying benefits.

- British social policy still assumes that women have the major role in child care. There is no state provision for paternity leave.
- Nursery education remains inadequately funded in the UK.
- The vast majority of child care is informal and organised in families or other groups. It is fragmented, generally inadequate and lags behind most EU countries.
- The lack of adequate child-care provision means that women are restricted to taking low-paid part-time work and continue to be caught in the poverty trap.
- Despite formal legislation on equal pay and equal opportunities there is still evidence to demonstrate women are disadvantaged in many aspects of life.
- Women as a group are most vulnerable to poverty when they are mothers, single and unsupported.
- Dependency, unpaid caring work, and erratic employment patterns renders many women vulnerable to poverty in old age.
- Policies on housing and homelessness are pro-natalist and assume that women are 'in the home' and that the household is of the 'male breadwinner' model.
- There is no evidence to support the myth that women become pregnant to gain access to housing.
- Social policies in which women are 'invisible' are outmoded and have been designed on the theories of the 'male breadwinner'.

Chapter 8

Power, professionalisation and midwifery

In this chapter we explore the nature of professionalisation and its significance and application for midwifery. We begin by looking at the sociological approach to a definition of a profession and at the way in which gender has been a crucial division of identity between the dominant male-based 'professions' and the largely female 'semi-professions' and at the strategies which different groups engage in order to construct spheres of power.

We then look at the social aspects of a profession and by using medicine as an example we look at the influence of social class, gender and ethnicity in the construction of this professional group. By focusing on the way in which the specialisation of gynaecology and obstetrics emerged and gained a place within the medical profession we analyse the way in which claims to a field of knowledge play a part in the creation of a 'profession'. This point is of great importance for a definition of midwifery as it has a claim to a specialised skill and the division between knowledge and skill or theory and practice, is one of the defining characteristics of a profession. We go on to look in more depth at the whole question and meaning of a 'skill', and ask, is this too a gendered concept?

This examination of the social meaning of a profession and the structures of power within which both doctors and midwives practice, includes a discussion on the impact of the Health Service reforms on the traditional hierarchies, especially with the advent of managerialism. The background to registration of midwives is discussed and the influence of the statutory bodies considered. The recent demands for separate legislation and a new Midwives Act are analysed. The chapter considers some aspects of the professional image of midwifery and the role of pressure groups and support networks. The final section considers some of the implications of social policy set out in *Changing Childbirth* (DOH, 1993). The chapter concludes with an analysis of a new power structure, managerialism.

■ What is a profession?

Why are some occupations such as medicine and the law regarded by society at large as professions, whereas others such as plumbing, hairdressing or taxi-driving are not? This is a question with which a branch of sociology has long been concerned. How does an occupation make itself recognised as a profession?

Traditionally within sociology, a definition of a profession has been arrived at through a 'trait' approach. This is the compilation of a set of characteristics and a group is defined as reaching the status of a profession if it meets the requirements of this checklist. Millerson (1964) collected a list of the most common traits of a model profession. These were:

- possession of skill based on theoretical knowledge;
- a long period of wide education and training;
- an altruistic notion of public service;
- a self-regulating code of ethics and conduct;
- the formation of a qualifying body which would decide on the competence of the membership.

In applying this approach it is possible to place an occupation upon a continuum stretching between an established profession, a marginal one and a new one. But this descriptive model does not address questions about the power exercised by professions nor the relationship between a profession and the social structure of a society.

Johnson (1972), introduced the notion of the professions as a means of controlling one's own working conditions and those of others. He argued that the characteristics of a profession act in the interests, not of society, but of the group itself. Therefore the so-called ethical strength and the altruism of dedication to public service, was, he argued, nothing more than an ideology. The public were placed in a position of subordination to the professional expert and had no means of challenge or resistance. Professionalisation was the means by which one occupation gained and exercised control over others and over the client group. One of the ways in which a group gained its status was through the ability to control entry to the professions. By thus controlling the supply of recruits the group could maintain a high price for its knowledge and could effectively control the labour market. The medical profession through the General Medical Council has been very successful in this means of control of entry and setting a market price for services (Ben-David, 1964)

A more Marxist-orientated approach to an analysis of the professions would be to relate the growth of professionalisation with a specific stage in industrial and welfare capitalism and also to look at the class membership of such groups.

Recent feminist approaches have stressed the gendered nature of the professions themselves and have argued that the whole value system of the professions is itself a masculinised one (Walby *et al.*, 1994; Witz, 1992;

Hearn, 1987). This approach has been especially apt in analysing the relationship between the professions and the designated semi-professions.

■ The semi-professions and women

The significance of gender in the definition of a profession was always obvious. But because the professions were almost exclusively male, the original sociological approach was to conclude that it was women themselves who lacked the necessary characteristics to gain admittance to a profession. Etzioni (1969), defined certain occupations as semi-professions and the defining characteristics of these were that they were occupations which existed within a bureaucratic structure and they were staffed mainly by women. The next step was to say that it was because women lacked sufficient authority and were too emotional, personal and subjective in their dealings with colleagues, that the occupations they performed could not qualify as a profession. This brought another dimension into a definition of professionalism: the necessity to be remote, to separate personal and professional judgements and to be objective, non-emotional and neutral. This, it was argued, effectively ruled out women because they were too taken up with trivial concerns about children and clothes to engage in serious objective discussion. Therefore the feminised semi-professions were ideal subordinates to the masculine professions as they accepted and indeed desired the role of 'handmaidens of a male occupation that has authority over them' (Simpson and Simpson, 1969 p. 231). In other words, as Anne Witz succinctly sums up, 'Because women are not men, the semi-professions are not professions' (Witz, 1992, p. 60). Jeff Hearn has argued (1987) that one of the roles of the feminised semi-professions is to take on the subjective and personal contact especially in emotional situations in the interaction with clients/patients and so enable the masculinised profession to keep its remote objectivity intact. In other words, it is the role of women as carers and handlers of emotion to intervene between a professional and a situation and so to deflect the grief and passion away from them.

In a Foucauldian analysis, space also plays a part in the representation of power structures in institutions. Access to the most powerful is always made difficult, the professional is not immediately available for consultation. Appointments have to be made, these are done through a subordinate and frequently an intermediary has to be seen first in order for the routine tasks to be carried out. A perfect example of this would be attendance at a hospital antenatal clinic. On entering any large organisation, a hospital, GPs' surgery, or a university, the first person encountered is of a low status – a porter, cleaner, receptionist – and then slowly progress is made until access to the professional is gained. In most buildings the actual siting of the offices follows the hierarchical pattern, with the top position the furthest away from the public.

The influence of gender upon definitions of a profession has been crucial and this is the reason why medicine as a masculinised profession and nursing and midwifery as feminised 'semi-professions' have been so much compared and studied. It is important to note that when we speak of medicine as a masculinised profession we do not just mean that men make up the vast majority of doctors (which is still true but changing) but also because the practices, work patterns and philosophies are taken to be masculine in influence. Before looking at the social structure of the medical profession as an example of a masculinised organisation, we now turn to an examination of the strategies employed by both dominant and subordinate groups.

■ Strategies of professionalisation

Anne Witz (1992) has characterised four main strategies which are employed by occupational groups in their battle to construct spheres of power and control. These strategies also demonstrate the over-determination of gender as well as other factors such as class and ethnicity in the composition of dominant and subordinate groups.

The model of strategies which Anne Witz has devised consist of four tactics, those of the dominant group are:

- *Exclusionary* The forcible exclusion of certain social groups from the occupation. An example of this would be the exclusion of women from medicine. Women were not allowed to attend universities to study and could not gain accreditation.
- *Demarcationary* This is the separation of another occupational or social group into a completely different sphere of practice over which the dominant group has control. The most perfect example of this is the separation of midwifery from obstetrics.

The successful completion by the dominant group of one or other or both of these tactics leaves the subordinate group with two means of resistance:

- *Inclusionary* This consists of the attempts by the excluded groups (women in medicine) to gain entrance via appeals to law or to the state. In medicine women were successful in some measure in this way although, as we shall see, that success is of a limited nature.
- *Dual closure* This refers to the acceptance of a group (midwifery) of a separate and subordinate status and the strategy of closure to prevent others from entering into it. For example, after the registration of midwives, the exclusion of unregistered ones and the unqualified. This

was also the practice in nursing where different grades, SEN and auxiliary, were created in order to keep the ranks of registered and qualified nurses intact. The strategy is twofold – the subordinate group attempts to gain a foothold in the dominant group and at the same time excludes others from entering. It is an example of countervailing power.

What becomes immediately obvious from a study of different groups is that the dominant ones are male-based and the subordinate ones are female. We will now move on to illustrate the ways in which this model of analysis can be applied both to the medical profession, to divisions within it and to the nature of the relationship between obstetrics and midwifery. It is important to remember that this is in the nature of an exercise in *analysis*, we are not merely describing 'what has happened', but are pointing to the overall model within which events and strategies can be understood.

■ The professionalisation of medicine

The medical profession which achieved professional status and increased power during the nineteenth century, has always been internally divided. Historically, medicine was made up of three separate groups; physicians, surgeons and apothecaries. From their inception these three groups mirrored the social class structure of the early nineteenth century. The physicians were Oxbridge- or Edinburgh-educated and often with a membership of the Church of England; they were regarded as 'gentlemen' and were the first to set up a Royal College to represent their interests. In the days when surgery was a very crude and often deadly business, surgeons were viewed as craftsmen or 'mechanics' and significantly they were originally represented by the Royal College of Barber-Surgeons, further illustrating their proletarian base. Surgeons originally were not qualified physicians and as such were addressed as 'Mr' and not 'doctor': this was insisted upon by the higher-status physicians. Apothecaries were shopkeepers and 'trade'. None of them really achieved the status of a profession until the Medical Act of 1858, which set up the General Medical Council to oversee and legitimise qualifications and to organise approved medical education. The role of the state was important here in the legitimising of medical education and recognised expertise. From then on, the medical profession increased in power and influence.

Throughout the nineteenth century the consultants became the élite of the profession, they were London based and exercised great authority over the newly set up teaching hospitals. General practitioners were seen as of a lower status and were those who had not enough money or influence to gain a consultants post and the apothecaries were slowly divorced from the profession and became a separate group. The division between consultants and general practitioners remained very strong and was an influence in the foundation of the NHS in 1948 (Honigsbaum, 1979). Even today, the advent of GP fundholding has been regarded by many as a means by which GPs have managed to gain a degree of control over consultants to whom they were traditionally subordinate. Until the NHS Act of 1948, consultants worked on a voluntary basis for a part of their time in the hospitals and then were free to practise privately for their livelihood. General practitioners had to buy a practice, which meant that practices in wealthier areas cost a great deal more than in deprived areas as of course they contained more patients who could afford to pay. Consequently many GPs were forced into competition with other, cheaper forms of health-care provision, the most notable being the competition over attendance at childbirth with midwives.

As well as this social division within medicine, there was the growth of specialisms, which led to a proliferation of consultants and attempts to legitimate diverse professional groupings. One such was obstetrics. The growth of medicine as a profession depended upon the development of theories of causation of diseases and more successful and scientifically based cures. The claim to professionalism was based upon a body of empirical scientific knowledge which informed successful practice. The advent of technological breakthroughs such as the microscope and anaesthetics further advanced not only the scientificity of medicine but its successful outcome. In ridding itself of the taint of medieval alchemy, magic and superstition, medicine achieved a professional status within a modern, rational, capitalist society. But there was an added significance to this professionalisation of a previous form of beliefs and practices: the gender of the practitioners also changed. The previous centuries had seen women as the 'natural' healers and community providers of cures and preventative measures. After 1858, the primary motivation of the medical profession was to make it exclusively male.

In her history of women doctors, Catriona Blake (1990) argues that when women tried to enter medicine they were seen as trying to *reclaim* their previous territory rather than to join a new occupation. The male medical profession resisted women's entry with a force which included physical abuse, verbal insults and violence. But most significantly the basis of the male domination of medicine was the siting of medical education and practice in the *public* sphere. Education could only be gained at universities, which did not admit women, very few women would have been taught Latin which was a prerequisite, and the Medical Registration Act itself specifically excluded women. The practice of medicine was also a market-based activity which involved a public presence and this further mitigated against women.

Much of this masculinisation of medicine was based upon a view of women which was given scientific validity by medical theories. Women's bodies were defined as inherently diseased, women were almost permanently 'unwell' and went from one biological crisis to another. It was further believed that all mental and emotional states were caused by their physiology and was centred upon the uterus. All female emotion was based here and the use of the Greek word 'hysteria' was synonymous with the word for womb. Feminist writers have pointed to the actual reality of women's lives in the nineteenth century to explain the supposed causes of female depression or mental illness, but before the development of psychology, the 'cure' for female emotional 'traumas' was often seen as surgery (Smith-Rosenberg, 1984). She argues that the removal of the clitoris was performed on some occasions to 'control' the sexual urges of a woman. It must be noted that for a woman to exhibit a sexual appetite was considered to be a form of mental derangement, hence the word 'nymphomania'. Given this deeply misogynist view of women, the idea of the presence of women themselves in a medical lecture room, or as colleagues in a hospital appeared as anathema to most medical 'men'. Another reason for the resistance to women, was that the financial rewards for the profession were still very precarious and it was feared that women would increase competition for a limited clientèle and it was feared that women would 'drag down' the profession to the status of nursing (Blake, 1990).

When women did finally qualify as doctors after the 1870s, they were invariably seen as providing a service to working-class and poor women. This can be seen as a demarcation tactic once inclusion had been gained. Many women doctors practised in women's infirmaries in slum areas and indeed there was evidence of a demand for women doctors from women themselves. The recent TV series, *Bramwell,* very accurately portrayed this early period. Today the majority of public health or community health doctors are women.

This occupation by a female occupational group or by females within a male occupational group has been termed by Witz (1992, p.5) as a *female professional* project. This refers to the attempts by women to keep separate their specific area of practice. A good example of this is radiography which historically women took over from men and which although occupying a subordinate position to radiology (male) nevertheless remained female-dominated (Witz, 1992). Another example would be the expansion of pharmacy as an academically based disciple, this became a female-dominated project after the 1960s. Within the claims made that a particular area is one in which either males or females have a special expertise, are appeals to 'naturalness'. Hence the role of midwives in 'normal labour'.

Although it would appear on the surface that the 'natural' sphere for women doctors would be in obstetrics and gynaecology and general practice, it was in these spheres that they received the greatest opposition. The professional ambitions of the medical profession were largely achieved, women even when admitted were kept out of high-status areas as were other social groups who were also perceived as 'outsiders'. What is the situation today in medicine for women and for ethnic minorities?

■ Medicine and social divisions

In 1995 60% of medical students in the UK were women. This signals a radical change from even the recent past when medical schools placed a quota on the numbers of women to be accepted. This practice was outlawed by the Sex Discrimination Act 1975. But does it signal an unequivocal victory for equality of opportunity? There is a number of related issues to be considered. First, the number of applications for places at medical school has declined dramatically in the past decade (they fell by 2.7% between 1985 and 1991). It is no longer a sought-after career for the traditional recruitment group of public-school boys. This decline in the popularity of medicine as a career is especially noticeable in general practice where the number of trainees has fallen to levels where some training courses have no candidates. Second, what are the promotional prospects for women once they qualify? Women still find it difficult to gain a consultancy post and they still represent under 20 per cent of all consultants and this is severely reduced in some specialities. One of the reasons for this is that appointments are still often made on the personal recommendation and social networks of senior consultants. Women do not 'belong' in this male world, they do not play rugby, probably did not go to the same school and are not 'one of the chaps', this is also true of people from the ethnic minorities.

In general practice where women are in most demand from female patients, the situation is still that of male-dominated partnerships with women making up the bulk of locum and part-time posts. General practice especially is based upon long hours and a commitment to night calls, neither of which is conducive to combining a family life with a professional one. Another example of the dominance of masculinised values and assumptions in a profession occurred in 1993. At a meeting of the Royal College of Physicians called to discuss the shortage of clinical researchers it was revealed that women faced great difficulty in getting accepted for accreditation despite the fact that they often had higher academic qualifications. The male establishment, it was reported (Smith, 1993, p. 6), was doubtful that women could gain a 'triple accreditation': that of clinician, scientist and mother'.

Has medicine managed to gain a social class mix in its recruitment patterns? A report in 1992 (Lowry, 1992, p. 1354) suggested that it had not changed in the past thirty years. The figures from UCCA showed that 38 per cent of students accepted were from the professional classes, whereas those from the skilled and unskilled manual class represented 0.7

per cent and 0.4 per cent of acceptances. The gender change has not therefore been reflected by a social class change and perhaps the middle-class male bias has been replaced by a middle-class female one.

In 1987 St George's Hospital Medical School was found to be discriminating against not only women applicants but those with a 'non-European sounding surnames' (CRE, 1988; Lowry and MacPherson, 1988). As a result of this revelation an ethnic monitoring of applicants and entrants to medical schools was enforced to prevent racial discrimination. What this revealed, however, was that there was a vast discrepancy of both application and acceptance between different ethnic groups. In Britain, students from an Asian background are overrepresented in ratio to the numbers in the population but those from Afro-Caribbean backgrounds remain underrepresented. It has been argued (MacManus *et al.*, 1990) that this reflects the different cultural ambitions of Asian families who encourage their children (especially boys) to gain universally recognised qualifications.

In a case which received great publicity in order to test hiring practices, two doctors sent identical applications for junior doctor posts but one was ostensibly from a white applicant and the other from an Asian one (Mason, 1995, p. 105). The resulting scandal was reported in the *British Medical Journal* (*BMJ*) (Smith, 1993) which supported their action and condemned the racism which was still obviously existing within the NHS. The reaction of the authorities was to arrest the doctors on charges of fraud, these were later dropped and the GMC found them not guilty of professional misconduct. But the case does highlight the informal racism which results in ethnic minority doctors (and women) being over-represented in the low-status specialisms such as geriatrics and psychiatry and underrepresented in posts in the high-status areas such as general surgery (McNaught, 1988, p. 40).

The fact that members of a social group which is perceived by the dominant one to be of lower status (ethnic minorities and women), are to be found in certain specialisms and not in others, begs the question as to why some areas of medicine achieved a higher status than others.

Becker (1977) argued that the hierarchy of specialisms within medicine followed the status placed upon the human body and its parts. In other words, the higher up the body the higher the prestige of the practitioner, brain surgeons occupying the top spot. Male bodies had a higher status than female ones, young bodies a higher status than old bodies and areas above the waist were seen as higher in status than those below. Therefore, those specialisms which were involved with elderly females would be of a lower status than those which were concerned with young males! Interestingly, psychiatry although dealing with the brain, is not a surgical or 'scientific' discipline, it does not therefore really 'belong' in the same category as neuro-surgery. This question of the cultural significance of specific medical specialisms is especially interesting in the development of gynaecology and obstetrics as a separate professional area of knowledge. The strategies employed by this particular occupational group, illustrate the argument of Dingwall and Lewis (1983) that professionalisation is the way in which a group tries to gain social mobility.

■ Professionalisation of gynaecology and obstetrics

As Ornella Moscucci (1990) has vividly chronicled, the professionalisation of gynaecology and obstetrics is a perfect example of the social mobility of an occupational group. The specialism had to:

- establish itself as a legitimate discipline,
- overcome opposition from established groups,
- gain social acceptance,
- demarcate the sphere of midwifery.

The binding together of gynaecology and obstetrics was an essential first step in the process of professionalisation. In the latter half of the nineteenth century, specialisms began to increase within medicine. Specialist hospitals were founded, mostly by doctors, as this was a way of establishing certain illnesses and conditions as requiring specialist treatment. Hospitals for women were founded at this time, based upon a Victorian ideal of femininity which required the 'delicate' middle-class woman to be treated with a degree of privacy and discernment. In these hospitals, pay beds were first introduced and patients would have been a cross-class mix of paying and 'charity' patients. The most famous of all the hospitals was the Chelsea founded in 1873 by James Aveling, an obstetrician and the founder of the British Gynaecological Society.

Gynaecology claimed to be the 'science of the whole woman', but bear in mind that all women's diseases were thought to be based upon her sexual organs. So any 'female disorder' was potentially within the province of gynaecology. Obstetrics and gynaecology were of course linked in many ways: the performing of a caesarian section and the controversial operation of ovariotomy were perceived as being almost similar as they both involved an abdominal sectioning which was within the province of surgery. With the development of anaesthetics, surgical interventions increased and the removal of the ovaries was now a feasible, if still highly dangerous, operation. But it was firmly situated within the realm of surgery and as such a new field of gynaecological surgery had to be constructed.

Ovariotomy was opposed by some of the medical profession because of its connotations of 'de-sexing' women and 'spaying'. One of the fiercest critics called surgeons who performed this operation 'belly rippers' (Moscucci, p. 153). But as the use of antiseptics grew, although notoriously slowly adopted by the British medical profession, the success rate of this operation improved and with it, its acceptability to the public and the medical profession. But its social respectability as a medical discipline took many years to achieve.

Gynaecology during its development in the Victorian era was the object of suspicion, opposition and had connotations with prostitution and pornography. Whilst obstetrics although connected to gynaecology had as its focus, childbirth and the achievement of motherhood, 'women's diseases' carried connotations of venereal infection.

This was evident during the 1860s when the Contagious Diseases Acts were passed. Various writers (Walkowitz, 1982; Hearn, 1992) have analysed the social meaning of these Acts within the patriarchal structure of state and medical legislation and practice. The Acts were designed to control the spread of venereal diseases and entailed the forcible inspection and incarceration of women who were suspected of being prostitutes in certain garrison and port towns. The Acts caused a great deal of political and feminist opposition as it was claimed that women were being treated like animals in order to protect male vice. The role of the medical profession in the inspection of women was one which caused a great deal of unease and suspicion in popular discourses.

For gynaecology, this opening-up of the debate on access to women's bodies by men was crucial to its professionalisation. The use of the speculum was the focus of much debate and concern. The 'steel penis' as it was often alluded to raised questions of the ownership of women's bodies, especially those of young unmarried women. In debates which recall those surrounding the employment of men-midwives, the propriety of males having physical knowledge of female 'patients' had to be assured. Opposition to the use of the speculum in gynaecological examinations came both from women themselves and from men uneasy about the aspect of the 'possession' of a woman by another man. Rape at this time was also the subject of much legal debate, and it was viewed as theft of virginity but it was the male 'owner', that is the father or guardian, who had been robbed. The gynaecological examination therefore must be seen against this background of the nineteenth century preoccupation with controlling sexual relationships within a male-headed family. The other problem for gynaecology was that it was associated not only with prostitution but with pornography. Judith Walkowitz (1992) has described how in Victorian pornographic texts, the occasion of the gynaecological examination was a frequent illustration and women were shown being tied down and 'speculumed' (Walkowitz, 1992, p. 99). The equipment of the gynaecologist, the riding master and the language of the hunting field were also connected. The use of the stirrups, in particular, evoked all three images much-used in pornographic literature. Interestingly, the case of Jack the Ripper which terrorised London in the 1880s was connected with the suspicion that 'Jack' was a doctor and knew about 'ripping-up' women (Walkowitz, 1982). The novel of *Dr Jekyll and Mr Hyde* also captured this popular suspicion about doctors, especially those who 'dealt' with women.

Gynaecology then had a difficult task in becoming a legitimate and respectable profession. By the end of the century, obstetricians on the staff of the specialist hospitals were becoming more skilled in ovariotomies and this operation was being more and more performed by them in these hospitals. In the general hospitals, however, the surgeons (who out-numbered obstetricians) retained the right to perform this operation. The battle between the two groups over the management of this procedure is described at length by Moscucci (1990). It was becoming increasingly clear to obstetric/gynaecologist surgeons that they had to define their own place in order to be recognised as teachers. Following the ban by surgeons, many obstetricians could not teach, as they did not have the necessary experience and knowledge of surgery.

Finally in 1929, the British College of Obstetrics and Gynaecology (it was not to be given the Royal accolade until 1945) was founded. It was the model illustration of an 'outsider' group which had finally legitimised its position. Not only was it an outsider in terms of the status of the specialism, its members were also of a lower social status.

Moscucci calls the founding of the College 'the provincial obstetricians' answer to the London gynaecological surgeons' (Moscucci, 1990, p. 184). The majority of both Fellows and Members were from the provinces or the 'white' colonies of Australia and South Africa. As with all other Colleges, women were in a very small minority. Fletcher-Shaw, one of the founders, explained the necessity of the connection between obstetrics and gynaecology: 'the primary object of the College is to bind obstetrics and gynaecology and to prevent gynaecology becoming a mere subdivision of surgery while obstetrics is left to those who have nothing better to do' (Moscucci, 1990, p. 184). From the foundation of the College in 1929 against the opposition of the other Royal Colleges, its progress was rapid. During the inter-war years when the concern over maternal mortality rates was receiving such publicity, the RCOG was in the forefront of plans and proposals for a national maternity service and was one of the leading advisory organisations in the setting-up of the National Health service after the war.

The hospitalisation of childbirth which accelerated after the foundation of the NHS also further institutionalised the demarcation of obstetrics and midwifery. The medical profession had always operated a demarcation strategy in respect of midwifery although this had not been a unanimous response. As Anne Witz has shown, there were two possible strategies which could have been used against midwifery:

• the strategy of de-skilling midwifery but preserving its status as an independent occupation;

- the strategy of ending the midwife's role altogether and replacing it with that of an obstetric nurse.

Although there was support for the latter alternative, the first strategy was the one which was enacted. One of the main reasons for this was that the sheer demand for midwifery services was too great for doctors to fulfil, many babies were born at night and also the poorer women who made up the clientèle of the midwife would not be able to afford to pay a doctor.

After the professionalisation of obstetrics and gynaecology as a group within the medical profession, the RCOG sought to demarcate roles of fellow-doctors further. After 1929, it moved to exclude GPs from membership of the College. In order to achieve this, postgraduate training and the sitting of an examination was required for membership. This was thought to discourage GPs who would not have the time to undergo training or study for examinations. After the foundation of the NHS, the RCOG also moved to exclude GPs from engaging in midwifery unless they possessed a specialist obstetric qualification. During the inter-war debates on the causes of maternal mortality it was largely GPs whom consultants blamed for unnecessary and inexpert interventions in childbirth. This strategy of excluding the competition from GPs in the management and control of childbirth was relatively successful. The hospitalisation of birth further cemented the control by obstetricians.

As far as the midwife was concerned, the Obstetrical Society in 1872 had set out the role for midwives, they were to be as 'the soldier is to the general' in the battle against maternal and child mortality in childbirth. This role was to remain, the medical profession was split over the licensing of midwives but, as we have seen, it finally adopted a 'de-skilling' approach to control and define the midwife's limitations in practice. But upon what basis did medicine and obstetrics claim to be a profession and midwifery a skill?

■ Theory and practice

There are two distinct threads of a debate on the occupational possession of an attribute such as knowledge or skill:

- there is the division between theory and practice which is far more than a mere difference in concept it is a *social division.*
- there is the definition of a skill – how does society define a skill and is its definition also a social one?

Theory and practice have historically been seen within the English culture as two separate spheres and also as belonging to two different social groups. The division within science between theoretical and applied science was illustrated throughout the English education system and was essentially a class division. The traditional and dominant view of the content of a university education was based firmly upon the classics- and humanities dominated Oxford and Cambridge. There was within this view a great resistance to science as a discipline and as early as 1830 Charles Babbage (the inventor of the original computer), in his report on the decline of science in England, criticised the public schools and ancient universities for their disregard of science (Cardwell, 1957). The dominant definition of an 'educated man' (women, of course, were not defined as such), which existed in the traditional sites of education was that of a 'man of letters', a person for whom knowledge was desirable for its own sake. It need not be 'practical' or 'useful' for the possessor of such knowledge would never actually need to earn a living through the application of useful knowledge. Even when Charles Darwin was attending Shrewsbury School in the middle of the nineteenth century there was no science on the curriculum and he was discouraged from his studies as they were not thought to be the 'proper' pursuit of a gentleman. When science was gradually introduced into the curriculum of the schools for the upper classes it was seen as an intellectual pursuit only. It was science as pure theory which was acceptable but not laboratory research which was defined as 'manual work' and, as such, more appropriate to the working class. As Lord Houghton wrote, 'For the solution of practical problems, the courier, the clerk or the plumber would always be available,' (Roderick and Stephenson, 1972).

Even by the 1880s it was calculated that science was taught in fewer than 20 per cent of public schools and to less than 10 per cent of the pupils. The entry of the middle classes into education altered the picture by the end of the nineteenth century with the founding of the Civic Universities in the large metropolitan areas which were based upon manufacturing. But the division between pure theoretical science and applied science remained strong. Pure abstracted theoretical science achieved a high cultural status slowly within the English culture but applied science, the practice of science, always remained of a lower status.

Medicine reflected this social class change. The majority of medical students came from the aspiring new middle class and therefore needed to earn a living but were also conscious of their need for social mobility. Medical students were regarded as a great deal 'rougher' than the students from the upper classes who were studying classics or literature, and this label remained until fairly recently. Medicine progressed from a practical-based activity to one which defined itself as a science and a theoretical as well as a practical activity. The need for theory was paramount, for without it, medicine would have remained merely a 'practice' which in terms of class and cultural status was more applicable to the skilled manual working class.

Many historians have chronicled the debates surrounding the

introduction of the teaching of science to the working classes (Barnes and Shapin, 1977). In the schools and Mechanics Institutes which were slowly being started for the education of the new industrial working class in the nineteenth century, scientific theory was either withheld or simplified. Science was only taught to the working class if it had been robbed of its questioning element and presented as a series of 'facts'. During this period, there was a great fear of revolution and science was seen as a radical and secular discipline which could encourage the working classes to revolution.

Many of the objections to the education of the working class remained couched in these terms into the present century. The idea was embedded in the English culture that the acquisition of skill and expertise was in some way a reflection of a 'natural' attribute and talent. Practice was 'natural', theory had to be taught and learned and so was therefore artificially gained. But the possession of 'practice' alone was a limit to the social mobility of the individual. The ambitious working-class mechanic needed to gain paper qualifications which would certify that 'he' also had a degree of theoretical knowledge. As the century progressed this emphasis on theory became more and more important in defining a skill and achieving professional status for an occupation. This historical and cultural definition of technical education as being of a lower status than a purely 'academic' one still exists today. The 'A' levels are held in higher regard than the vocational qualifications; grammar schools for the 'academic' child are of higher status than technical colleges and places in British universities to do applied sciences remain unfilled. In this cultural structure of the emphasis on the academic as opposed to the technical, to theory as opposed to practice, occupations which previously conducted their 'training' within their own institutions or 'on the job' have now moved into the sphere of higher education. Notable among these are the health and social care professions, especially midwifery, nursing and social work.

How can we understand these moves? It could be interpreted as a rational judgement on behalf of the occupation that in order to achieve a professional status they must be placed within the site of the traditional purveyors of abstract theory and of *education* rather than *training*. For it is the possession of a theory which is an essential ingredient for professionalisation. Interestingly, within universities themselves there has been opposition to the entry of such disciplines on the grounds that they do not 'belong' as they are vocational and practice-based.

But this move to acquire a theoretical connection to a practice is not without its critics among the ranks of supporters of the aspiring professions. Many of the criticisms are reminiscent of those of the nineteenth century when it was proposed that the working class did not need education as it possessed a 'natural' talent for mechanical engineering.

One such critic of the moves within midwifery education to construct a theoretically based practice, is Marjorie Tew (1995). She has long been an opponent of the medicalisation of childbirth and of the professionalisation of obstetrics and the 'deskilling' of midwifery and so therefore her critique of this move must be addressed in detail.

> She wrote: It would be a mistake to imagine that a successful academic, an expert in theory, is necessarily a successful midwife ... [the profession] must not let itself be educated out of its appreciation of the overriding importance of positive emotions and basic good health in the mother by teachers whose untested scientific theories may fail to fit the facts. (p. 77)

This is an extraordinary set of comments and ideological assumptions which contain many of the antagonisms which accompanied the upper-class rejection of the education of the working classes last century. The division of theory and practice is maintained by Tew as is the belief that all a good midwife needs is a 'natural' aptitude for caring and common sense. This downgrading of education and academic thought is characteristic of those who would wish to 'de-professionalise' such occupations as midwifery, nursing, teaching and medicine. We will discuss this move within health policies later in this chapter. The logical outcome of such a move against higher education in midwifery would be to set the requirement for entry as being a 'sensible, and good woman', which for midwifery would be a step which would take it back to the pre-registration period. As Ros Bryar (1995, p. 202) has so clearly explained, it is only through the rigorous process of identifying concepts, building and testing theories, scientific or otherwise, that midwifery care can develop.

We have established that one of the necessary qualifications for professionalisation is the acquisition of a body of theoretical knowledge which can inform practice. This theory-based practice is then perceived as a *universal* qualification rather than a personal attribute based upon *individual* experience and observation. Midwifery is aspiring to this goal as we shall see in the following discussion but before we move on to look at midwifery organisation and education, let us consider the concept of *skill*.

■ What is skill?

The most important factor in the comparison of midwifery and engineering in terms of its perception as a practice and a skill, which contained 'natural' attributes and did not therefore need the input of education is, of course, gender.

Many writers (Cockburn, 1980, 1985; Crompton and Sanderson, 1990), have argued that the category of skill is a gender-based one and is not related in any objective way to the tasks performed. In other words, activities performed by men are categorised as skilled whereas the same or similar activities performed by women are defined as unskilled or at best, semi-skilled. Sylvia Walby (1990) has analysed this situation as one which takes place within the patriarchal structures of most work organisations. In Britain, as in most other countries, the labour market is characterised by both vertical and horizontal segregation of men and women. That is to say that most men work in separate industries and spheres from women and they mostly work with other men. Men and women each tend therefore to work with their own sex, which makes claims for equal pay difficult to sustain as we saw in Chapter 7.

This gender segregation allows the tasks performed within occupations to be labelled as skilled or unskilled dependent upon whether they are performed by women or men. Catherine Hakim (1979) showed examples of this in the paper-box industry, where the same tasks were defined differently depending upon the gender of the worker. This differential definition of skill is, of course, crucial in setting pay rates and status.

Many of the tasks performed by women in the labour force stem from the *private* sphere of the home, and so even if performed in *public* for money they are still regarded as 'women's work' and therefore defined as unskilled and poorly rewarded. Conversely, there are few tasks which are seen as 'men's work' in the private sphere of the home – electrical maintenance, plumbing, and possibly building – but these are not applicable to all men and they carry far greater public rewards than do child-care or cleaning.

This definition of the skills appropriate to men and women also carry connotations of being 'natural' attributes. Within the dominant cultural view, women are said to be 'naturally' suited to caring, they are more careful and conscientious, and physically they have more manual dexterity. These beliefs then become concretised into the types of work which women perform in the labour market. The advent of technology has reinforced many of these views rather than overturned them. In her study of the microwave industry, Cynthia Cockburn (1993, p. 45) gave a vivid illustration of the gender ideologies at work, in the words of a (male) manager, women were suitable for the 'fiddly' jobs where you could 'get your fingers in there', and also were more able to cope with routine and boring jobs which required periods of inactivity, whereas the men required action and control over the processes.

This scenario could be used to sum up the division between the medical profession and midwifery in the control and management of the birth process. In their strategy of demarcation, the medical profession assigned to midwives the control of 'normal' births, which required little action and involved periods of waiting and watching. This was one of the reasons why many GPs were relieved to relinquish attendance at births in the post-war period, because of their time-consuming and 'non-essential' nature.

In the demarcation strategy employed by the medical profession was the redefinition of the midwives' skill, the ability to recognise her limitations. Midwives were required to recognise impending abnormalities and to refer to the 'expertise' of the doctor. How skilled were midwives? As Moscucci (1990) records, this is historically vague. Certainly there were many who were highly skilled and talented and who pioneered many new techniques, but there must also have been a number who did not possess talent or ability. But midwifery as a whole, it is often claimed was 'de-skilled' with the development of birth technology and the medicalisation of childbirth.

There are alternative views to this. Dingwall *et al.* (1988) suggest that in fact midwifery was 're-skilled' rather than 'de-skilled' by technological developments. The process of 'de-skilling' is one which the Marxist writer Braverman (1974) argues is a structural process in capitalist development which has the ultimate objective of reducing all labour to an unskilled status.

Midwifery nevertheless is constant in its definition of midwifery practice as a skill. It is the *skill* of the midwife which it is claimed has consistently been under-used and downgraded and which the new *Changing Childbirth* proposals are aimed to reinstate. But as we have seen skill is not an unambiguous concept, skill is both gender- and class-based. The claim to possess a specialised *skill* is not the mark of a profession but of a craft. Is midwifery then redefining itself as a craft rather than aiming for full and unequivocal recognition as a profession? As we shall see later in this chapter, the new organisational reforms within the NHS may make this a rational strategy. Instead of operating the strategy of usurpation, perhaps midwifery should engage in the strategy of a craft project.

We now turn to look in detail at the organisation and position of midwifery itself.

■ The professionalisation of midwifery

□ The past

The midwives' path to professional status has been long and fraught. They were acclaimed and respected in ancient Greece; valued, well-established in Rome, and yet burnt at the stake as witches in medieval Britain (Ehrenreich and English, 1973). Along the way nurses and doctors have been both friends and enemies.

The history of midwifery has been described and discussed in detail by many authors. Towler and Bramell trace the history and consequences in 'Midwives in History and Society' (1986), whilst Jean Donnison's book *Midwives and Medical Men* is a history of the struggle for the control of childbirth. Most recently Leap and Hunter (1993) have published their oral history of midwifery in *The Midwife's Tale*. All the histories trace the move from handywoman or 'the woman you sent for' to the professionalised midwife. Midwives are mentioned in the Bible and all through history but evidence of incompetence in the birth attendants emerged in the late nineteenth century. According to Arney (1992) male midwives appeared in the seventeenth century. In 1892 a select Committee Report on Midwives' Registration, confirmed that the practice of many untrained 'handywomen' left a lot to be desired. Some handywomen trained as apprentices with some formal theoretical instruction, but many others were self-trained or untrained. Their services were free or very cheap. Some women offered a gift or donation. The medical profession, anxious to participate in or according to some authors, control childbirth, were alarmed at the poor standards but unwilling to intervene in cases where there was no likelihood of payment. Gradually more men became involved in birth and their higher status and the use of forceps led to their position and power. But midwives were on the road to respectability and status (Hunt and Symonds, 1995). As a result of intensive activities by pressure groups (Towler and Bramall, 1986) and the sterling work of individuals such as Dame Rosalind Paget, as well as the changing political climate of the day, the Registration of Midwives Act 1902 was passed. At first the members of the 'Midwives' Institute' were prepared to support proposals that placed the new Central Midwives Board under the control of the General Medical Council. It was the Manchester Midwives Society that argued that 'no registration' was preferable to registration under medical domination. (Donnison, 1988, pp. 140–59). The 1902 Act achieved the elimination of the undesirable 'handywoman' and the creation of a legitimate register. The move to a state-salaried service was completed in 1936 with the passing of the 1936 Midwives Act.

In 1903 midwifery training lasted three months and extended to six months in 1923 for those already nurses and one year for non nurses. In 1938 the two-part training was introduced and the length extended to one year for nurses and two years for non-nurses (Towler and Bramall, 1986). The Central Midwives' Board set up in 1902 increased its membership from the original nine to fourteen and then to sixteen places. In 1983 midwifery training was increased to eighteen months for nurses and to three years for non-nurses.

□ **The statutory bodies**

In 1970 a committee, under the Chairmanship of Professor Asa Briggs was set up to: 'Review the role of the nurse and the midwife in hospital and community and the education and training required for that role, so that the best use is made of available manpower to meet present needs and the needs of an integrated health service'. The committee had twenty members, but just one was a practising midwife (RCM, 1991). The committee reported in October 1972 and its findings had far reaching implications for the future of midwifery education and practice. Amongst its main recommendations was for a five-body statutory framework, the United Kingdom Central Council for Nursing, Midwifery and Health Visiting (UKCC) and the four National Boards. It claimed to recognise the real and important differences between nursing and midwifery' and later concluded that there are aspects of midwifery on which a body dealing also with all aspects of nursing could not rightly pronounce with necessary authority (RCM, 1991). This statement probably led to the establishment of a standing midwifery committee at the UKCC and the National Boards. But the recommendations of the Briggs committee were not accepted wholeheartedly by all midwives. The Central Midwives Board thought the structure of the Council and separate boards would diminish and fragment control of the midwifery profession. Many midwives rejected the carrot of self-regulation saying that midwifery was in danger of exchanging medical dominance for control and rule by nurses.

In 1979 the Nurses, Midwives and Health Visitors Act was passed and in 1983 the control of midwifery education and practice passed to the UKCC and to the National Boards in each of the four countries. The underlying principles of the Act were, first, regulation of practice for the protection of the public, and second, government of the three professions, by the professions, for the professions.

The functions of the UKCC were set out in the Act. These are to define and set standards for education and practice and through the professional conduct system improve professional conduct. The UKCC maintains a single professional register and has a role in international matters including compliance with relevant EU Directives.

The National Boards in each of the four countries is required to collaborate with the UKCC, award qualifications and issue advice and guidance to Local Supervising Authorities. The Boards' main function is to approve educational institutions and courses and to ensure that courses meet the UKCC standards for registration.

In 1989 a firm of management consultants, Peat, Marwick & McLintock, were appointed by the government to review the statutory body structure. The report published in 1989 found that the 1979 Act was cumbersome, excessively bureaucratic. Decision-making was lengthy and the report recommended that the body to set the standards for the profession should also be the elected body. In 1992 an Act to amend the 1979 Act was passed. This Act changed the shape of the Boards and Council and probably strengthened the position of the UKCC. The Council became the elected body and its membership increased from 45 to 60. Two-thirds of the membership are elected and one-third appointed by the Secretary of State. It was strongly argued that in order to fulfil its function the UKCC needed such a large membership, not least because of the work of the Professional Conduct Committee which at that time was still dealing with a backlog of cases. The delays were sometimes as long as two years between reporting an alleged offence and a committee hearing. The professions elected the new Council which included ten members from each country and twenty appointed members. There are two midwife members from each of the four countries. The investigation of alleged professional misconduct became the responsibility of the UKCC instead of the National Boards. The Midwifery section of the 1992 Act removed the UKCC's requirement to consult with the National Boards on midwifery matters, although in practice they still do on some issues. The amendments also gave the Council the right to prescribe standards with respect to advice and guidance on supervision. This impinges on the Boards' responsibilities and places the UKCC in more of a watchdog position.

The structure of the National Boards changed with the Chairman being appointed rather than elected by the membership. The Boards also include a number of members appointed by the Secretary of State. The Chairman must be a nurse, midwife or health visitor and appointments include individuals appointed by virtue of their qualifications in nursing, midwifery or health visiting. There is a Chief Executive, other executive members and other officers. The National Boards were no longer obliged to have any Standing Committees and indeed all four have chosen other methods of obtaining midwifery advice.

The new statutory body structures mirror the format of Health Authorities and Trusts. They are certainly smaller with clearly defined responsibilities and powers. It is also clear that the democracy evident in the 1979 Act has diminished and it is more difficult to argue that there is still government of the professions, by the professions, for the professions.

☐ **The present, a call for a new Midwives Act**

For many years, certainly since the 1979 Act, a growing number of midwives have expressed dissatisfaction with the present statutory body framework. The Association of Radical Midwives (ARM) founded in 1976 were very concerned that the unique and separate nature of the midwifery profession would be compromised by the new bodies. The cry to 'bring back the CMB' was commonly heard at ARM meetings. The case of Jilly Rosser who was removed from the Register for professional misconduct and subsequently reinstated on appeal (*Daily Telegraph*, 25 February 1989) further fuelled the demands for separate legislation. In 1991 the ARM produced a 'Midwifery Legislation Group Manifesto'. The document argued that since the passage of the 1979 Act 'the midwifery profession has seen further erosion of its autonomy and is experiencing difficulties in meeting the needs of childbearing women'. They argued that amalgamation with a numerically stronger profession (nursing) has resulted in midwives spending most of their time defending their profession. In 1990 the English National Board and later the Welsh National Board decided to reorganise the professional-advisor role so that advisors had a more generic role. In England the advice of the Midwifery Committee was ignored (Jackson, 1993) whilst in Wales the Midwifery Committee was not even consulted (Hunt, 1993). On that occasion the Chairman of the WNB believed that the issue being considered was an internal management issue and not a 'midwifery issue'. A 'midwifery issue' is not defined in statute, thus, if the majority of the Board who are nurses, define a midwifery issue, then on occasions the opportunity even to offer advice is subsequently lost. The National Boards were not even obliged to take the Midwifery Committee's advice but the position at UKCC is somewhat stronger. Section 4(4) of the 1979 Act states that the Secretary of State should not approve rules relating to midwifery unless he or she is satisfied that they have been framed in accordance with the recommendations of the midwifery committee. This of course presumes that there is agreement on what is a midwifery issue and that it is a concern likely to be resolved by midwives' rules.

In 1990 at the RCM Annual Conference the branch delegates' meeting voted to support a campaign for new legislation. The Council of the RCM chose to set up a commission to review the Act and its implications for the profession. The commission was chaired by Lady Wyndham Kaye. The commission, financially and administratively supported by the RCM but independent, published its findings in July 1991 (RCM, 1991). It concluded that the available evidence clearly shows that the weaknesses in the Act are 'neither resolvable, nor of such magnitude as to make a campaign for a new Act either practicable at the present time nor yet proved to be desirable'.

Subsequently and during consultations on the review of the statutory bodies by the management consultants, Peat, Marwick & McLintock (1989), the RCM lobbied the UK Chief Nurses, the Chairman and Chief Executive of the five statutory bodies to make necessary amendments to the Act. The RCM then established 'Legislation Watch' to monitor the 1992 Act.

In 1995, again at the RCM Annual Conference, the issue came to the forefront again. Once again midwives called for separate legislation. Again the vote was won. The press reports proclaimed that 'Midwives prepare to go it alone'. Not everyone agreed (Hunt, 1995) but the issue has been reopened.

The arguments and passions for a new Midwives' Act are inextricably linked with midwives' autonomy and independence. As explained in Chapter 4 the role of the midwife has changed with the hospitalisation and medicalisation of birth. In the past, midwives had their own statutory body, the Central Midwives Board, and were largely independent practitioners giving care throughout pregnancy, labour and the puerperium. As birth in hospital became the norm midwives became contributors to systems of fragmented care. Despite efforts to make better use of midwives' skills in many government reports (Maternity Services Committee 1980 and 1984: *Short Report*) little has so far changed. But the framework is in place to reinstate midwives' autonomy (House of Commons, 1992; DOH, 1993) and with this change in the status and position of midwives a new Act may prove to be appropriate. Much will depend on midwives' willingness to resume their former responsibilities and accept accountability for their actions. Most midwives in Britain have still trained first as nurses and are more familiar with the role as helper in care than leader of care.

■ Professional regulation and covert control

There is an argument that professional regulation is more about protecting the professions than the apparently altruistic function of protecting the public. As we have already seen earlier in this chapter Johnson (1972) argues that professions exist as a means of controlling working conditions and that the characteristics of a profession act for the well-being, not of society, but of the group itself.

The arguments for and against the form of statutory control will no doubt continue. But deregulation also appears to be on the present government's agenda. It is seen as economical and effective. As midwives argue over a separate act, other bodies with regulating functions, e.g. The National Council for Vocational Qualifications are waiting in the wings.

Sometimes the statutory bodies are criticised for exerting too much control. Jenkins (1995) asks, 'What other profession has a set of Rules that prescribed in law the need to keep records and to open practice premises for inspection, and a duty to be medically examined and to be supervised?' She considers that the time when the Central Midwives Board were in control was the time of the gradual decline in midwives' autonomy. This of course excludes at least one other contributing factor, the medicalisation and hospitalisation of birth. She would like to see future regulation not only protecting women but also allowing midwives to function as autonomous practitioners.

■ Midwifery education

The Midwives' Rules (UKCC, 1993) set out the standards for midwifery education and the word 'training' was removed. For registered nurses the course lasts for 80 weeks, and takes three years for non-nurses. Since 1995 both courses are referred to as either 'Pre Registration Midwifery Education' or 'Pre-Registration Midwifery Education (Shortened)' both courses lead to registration on Part 10 of the UKCC Register and must also lead to an academic qualification no less than a Diploma in Higher Education. The entry requirements are still five subjects at GCSE and must include English and a science subject. There are many other courses now approved as alternative entry qualifications, e.g. Access courses, BTEC and more recently NVQ. Grave predictions about a 'demographic time bomb' set to explode in 1995 appear to have been exaggerated. There are no shortages of either qualified midwives or potential new recruits. The prolonged and deep economic recession, combined with the total overhaul of the NHS and the move to a market-orientated economy may be contributing factors.

The Rules state that programmes of education must be conducted at approved educational institutions (validated by a National Board) and that those undertaking the three-year course will have 'supernumerary status'. This concession together with the payment of bursaries rather than salaries to student midwives was achieved as part of the legislation that introduced the Project 2000 courses for student nurses. Student midwives undertaking the shortened course are salaried and are still expected to contribute rostered service throughout their course.

The student must be directed throughout the course by the approved educational institution as opposed to clinical service managers, and must include periods of practical experience in midwifery. The outcomes of the programmes are defined and set out in the rules. The programmes must meet the requirements of the EC Midwives Directives and enable the student, once qualified, to function competently and safely as a midwife.

There has been a distinct change of emphasis in midwifery education with more attention being paid to academic qualifications. Research is a key area and students are taught to appreciate and be critical of research evidence and to evaluate practices in maternity care. Continuing education programmes are well-established but more and more midwives are finding difficulty in securing financial support from their employers. Diploma courses are run part-time, during the evenings and at weekends to accommodate the needs of qualified midwives. The first Professors of Midwifery have been appointed and courses leading to Bachelors and Masters courses are well-established in many areas. The UKCC requirements for Post-Registration Education and Practice have encouraged more and more midwives to return to some level of formal continuing education. (UKCC 1990, 1993). Naturally there has been some resistance to this move to an academic status. Many midwives are anxious and threatened by change and the medical profession itself is not without its words of caution including Marjorie Tew whose comments are discussed earlier in this chapter, under the heading 'Theory and Practice'.

The pursuit of scholarship is likely to be the key to improving practice; whilst there is little supporting evidence available, this belief certainly has the support of the statutory bodies and central government.

But there are other issues of concern in midwifery education. As the curriculum has broadened and lengthened, teachers other than midwives have become involved in midwifery education. As this book testifies, experts in sociology, social policy, psychology, law, ethics, and the biological sciences now make a valuable contribution to midwifery education. At the same time there has been reduction in the demand for newly trained midwives. The recession as well as changes in the health service have also led to fewer midwives being trained. As a consequence many midwife teachers have lost their jobs and some blame the statutory bodies. Minor changes in approval criteria such as the move away from Student–Teacher Ratios (STRs) are blamed for loss of midwifery education posts (Roch, 1995). The other major concern is that as midwifery moves in to universities and other higher education establishments midwifery will lose control of its education. When curriculum heads who are not midwives manage midwifery education programmes, the step towards midwifery becoming merely a branch of the bigger, dominating profession of nursing becomes more likely. This concern, along with others, has prompted the UKCC to issue a Registrar's letter (8/94) in which it states that all midwifery programmes 'must demonstrate midwifery content and application throughout the total duration of the course'. This effectively prevents any College from offering any kind of midwifery course based on the nurses' Common Foundation Programme and a subsequent midwifery branch programme.

But the pressures on midwifery educationalists as small fish in an increasingly large pond are mounting. It is becoming more and more difficult to protect and safeguard the unique identity of midwifery, the onus of responsibility rests with senior midwifery educationalists with support and guidance from statutory bodies and professional organisations that have the interests of midwives at heart.

The move into higher education has brought many advantages, not least the increased resources, access to better libraries and intellectual stimulation and creative opportunities (Hunt, 1993a). The disadvantages are the increasing difficulties of maintaining links with clinical areas and clinical competence in the competitive world of higher education.

■ What is a midwife? Public images and reality

The public image of midwifery is confused. According to Hunt (1995) 'Midwives are frequently referred to as 'nurse' and the public perception is a misty mix of elderly matrons in ancient Morris Minors and high technology intensive care nurses in trouser suits.'

For more than two generations midwives have worked predominantly in hospitals. Community midwives are seen to be mainly concerned with post-natal care and are often confused with Health Visitors. The hospital midwife has assumed the role of doctor's assistant and with it the title of nurse. The medical model of care (see also Chapter 4) is now so firmly entrenched in the minds of midwives, doctors and women that any other title is inappropriate. Obstetric practice has been described as reductionist, anti-feminist and interventionist (Chalmers *et al.*, 1980). Bryar (1995) argues that 'many midwives would agree that the influence of the medical model is so pervasive in society and in health care organisations that it has to be recognised, faced and addressed before any discussion can be held about any other model of midwifery practice'. Hence midwives and their image are part of a society that believes that birth is an illness, to be treated in hospital, by a doctor assisted by a nurse who has specialised in a branch of nursing called 'midwifery'!

The case for a separate pay structure for midwives has been argued year after year by the Royal College of Midwives and appears to have been won in 1995. This argument has been rejected year after year by nurses who believe that midwifery is no more than a specialist branch of nursing.

■ Pressure groups and other influences

Pressure groups in the maternity services have appeared mainly in response to the medicalisation of birth. Some groups have a distinctly political message in that they exist to change government thinking and social policy whilst other groups are pressure groups but also have a function in offering information and support to individuals and groups. The MIDIRS 'Directory of Maternity Organisations' 1989 lists 163 different organisations that are connected in some way with the maternity services. They include The Association for Post-Natal Illness, Birth works (arranges hire of tubs for water birth), Caesarean section Support Group, Child Poverty Action Group, Down's Syndrome Association, Episiotomy Support Group, Foundation for the Study of Infant Deaths, Health Rights, International Home Birth Movement, The Pre-eclamptic Toxaemia Society (PETS). This list goes on and on.

All these groups function in a democracy as advocates for the people and aim to inform and improve a particular aspect of maternity care. The three best-known groups are the National Childbirth Trust (NCT) and the Association for the Improvements in Maternity Services (AIMS) and the Maternity Alliance established in 1980 and which is concerned with inequality, poverty and the benefits system.

Durward and Evans (1990) explore the key functions of pressure groups as advocacy agencies. They state the four functions of advocacy as

- personal
- professional
- public
- practical

and go on to explain how the priorities of particular groups determine the balance of these advocacy roles and the sectors they serve.

How do midwives see such groups? There is evidence (Hunt and Symonds, 1995) that some midwives are disparaging about the contribution made by some organisations. The NCT seems to come in for particular criticism in that the organisation is perceived as offering women unrealistic expectations of birth. There is evidence that some midwives feel that their professional integrity is in some way threatened by 'amateurs' i.e. not professionals, but those whose knowledge has been acquired by experience not training and who are able to offer appropriate advice. Yet many midwives acknowledge the contribution made by breast-feeding counsellors and by women who work with women with post-natal depression.

It appears that while midwives should value and acknowledge the contribution that pressure groups make in changing policy they should be wary of involving an army of unpaid voluntary carers in maternity care. The case for housekeeping support has been well made (Flint, 1994) but arrangements for maternity care must remain within the statutory provision of health care.

■ *Changing Childbirth*: some implications of social policy

Changing Childbirth is the Government's (DOH) response to the House of Commons Health Committee Report on Maternity Services (HOC, 1992) in England. In Wales – and somewhat earlier (August 1991) – the Welsh Health Planning Forum released its Protocol for Investment in Health Gain for Maternal and Child Health and this set as a target that 50 per cent of all mothers should have access to a scheme offering continuity of care by 1997, and that by 1993 60 per cent of women should describe pregnancy and childbirth as a positive experience.

The Welsh Office is committed to a goal of continuity of care but has failed to endorse *Changing Childbirth* and its target or accept it as policy for the NHS in Wales. One can only speculate as to the reasons for this resistance and maybe the medical profession has again used its power to prevent a total commitment to choice and home birth. The Protocol document is in the process of review under the auspices of the Directors of Public Health Medicine.

More recently the document, *Caring for the Future*, has been released and there is still the aim of continuity of care in maternity services. In Northern Ireland, a Maternity Unit Study Group was established by the Department of Health and Social Services in October 1993 to consider the potential for extending the range of options of care available to women during childbirth through the development of units led by midwives and/or general practitioners. The report *Delivering Choice* was produced in 1994. In Scotland a policy review of the provision of maternity services was carried out in 1993 and the recommendations are being taken forward by a Framework for Action Working Group of the Clinical Resources and Audit Group/Scottish Health Management Efficiency Group (CRAG/SCOTMEG). In all four countries there is a commitment to increasing choice in childbirth and to improving continuity of carer.

Changing Childbirth is the clearest and most positive document and its aims are being supported by substantial funds from the Department of Health, but these funds are only available for use in England. There is no doubt that without exactly recommending a move to home birth, the emphasis has shifted firmly towards the woman's right to choose. It can be argued that the whole idea of a choice is part of the new market economy in health care. Customers in any sort of market need choice.

But what are the implications of such a change in policy? In 1993 the Royal College of Midwives commissioned the Institute of Manpower Studies to undertake a study called 'Developing Continuity of Care in Maternity Services' (Stock and Wraight, 1993). The researchers were especially interested in the implications for midwives. The study included five case studies from units where schemes were in place. The authors concluded that there were advantages and disadvantages to such schemes. The advantages included greater job satisfaction for midwives but there were difficulties in developing systems that did not result in midwives working excessive hours. Some midwives anticipated difficulties in fitting new working patterns into part-time work and around their existing personal needs and commitments. There was little evidence to suggest that teams were more expensive and good evidence of enhanced care to women and their families. Continuity depended to a great extent on the number of midwives in the teams and certainly team midwifery did not suit all midwives. The authors conclude that team midwifery is in its infancy and is not a panacea for all the problems associated with providing continuity of care.

There is certainly anecdotal evidence and concerns about 'burnt-out midwives' (Sandall, 1995) who are attempting to offer continuity of carer. Teams, when well-planned seem to offer midwives support. But midwives working alone or in groups of two or three find the ideal of continuity of carer too demanding. Some writers are warning that both women and midwives may have higher expectations of the maternity services than can yet be achieved (Warwick, 1995).

Time will show the impact of this social policy on women, their families and on midwives. Case loads may be the answer for some women and some midwives in some areas but it is more likely that a variety of schemes designed to meet the unique needs of different areas are more likely to emerge. There is a grave danger in any new and complex change that the leaders and the followers may lose sight of the original vision. *Changing Childbirth* was about improving the quality of the birth experience for women. It focused on improving communication, to improve feelings of control and to help women with the decisions around childbirth. It was not about off-duty rotas, on-call systems and teams. These are important, but not as important as listening to what women want and need in their experience of childbirth.

■ New power for old?

In this chapter we have been concerned with the professionalising strategies of both medicine and midwifery, but there is another ingredient in this analysis of power, the advent of a new power structure: managerialism.

Managerialism is so called because it is an ideology which sets up a new relationship between the organisation itself and its aims and objectives. It is a paradigm of a way of organising structures in order to produce efficiency. Managerialism denotes an objective means of producing efficiency without hindrance from traditional hierarchies. In a way it is the opposite to professionalism with its specialities and bodies of exclusive knowledge; managerialism is based upon the *application* of techniques rather than purely scientific quest for knowledge. Managerialism is not concerned with demarcation of responsibilities and spheres of control, as are professions, but with the direction of the whole operation.

After 1974, the NHS had been reorganised and power had been decentralised with management teams set up in each district. It was under this early reorganisation that nursing gained much in terms of status and a hierarchical presence on management boards. But the emphasis was on a system of consensus management which had no direct chain of command. Although as Strong and Robinson (1990) illustrate many of the traditional hierarchical relationships between nursing (and presumably midwifery) and medicine remained intact, there was a degree of power which was fragmented between the occupational groups. The system however was characterised by 'medical individualism and nursing subordination' (Strong and Robinson, 1990, p. 41).

In 1980, this lack of a command structure was focused upon by the incoming government as one of the main stumbling blocks to the achievement of the three 'E's; efficiency, economy and effectiveness. The internal structures and power groupings of the professions with their demarcatory strategies were also seen as remnants of an old system which were standing in the way of the implementation of a new Health Service. In many ways a new managerialist input was seen as the way to overcome these traditional structures and to implement the new reforms of the organisation.

The philosophy which underpinned the policies of the Thatcher administration was that of changing the public sector from a profession-dominated bureaucratic paternalism which they believed typified the whole of the post-war welfare state and nationalised industries. This signalled a whole new set of relationships to be set up between the 'old' patients or clients of the professionals and the 'new' consumers who were to be given choice and were encouraged to demand higher standards of service.

In 1983, the government commissioned a management survey of the NHS, headed by Sir Roy Griffiths who had proved his 'skill' and expertise in the management of Sainsbury's, the successful supermarket chain. The object was to transpose the values of entrepreneurial management from a successful private and market-based business to the public sector. The subsequent Griffiths Report (1983) identified the lack of a direct line of control in the NHS. This was summed up in the phrase, 'If Florence Nightingale was carrying her lamp through the corridors of the NHS today, she would almost certainly be searching for the people in charge' (Griffiths, 1983, p. 12).

This statement is very revealing in that it presumes that the 'people in charge' will not be nurses! The subsequent management reforms of the 1980s and 1990s bore out this assumption. Although managerialism has a genderless label, nevertheless it still embodies many of the traditional ideologies of the 'natural' attributes of men and women. The new style of management was often called 'macho', which relied upon the obvious show of strength and a threatening and even bullying approach, which was not easy for women to adopt. But as Jane Newman (1995) suggests, managerialism as a 'transitional' culture often opened up occupational spaces for women. Women managers often adopted a more 'traditional' approach – that of 'mothering' or being a 'bossy aunt' or even using flirting to control male subordinates. But within management structures women and men tend also to be gender segregated. Finance management which is the higher status is nearly always occupied by men whereas personnel or 'people' management is the female sphere.

Management control over the medical profession tended to be limiting of the expenditure on treatments and surgery, so that the always existing rationing of care which had been practised unofficially by doctors (Harrison and Pollitt, 1994) now became a strategy of management control.

The other parallel move to reorganise the Health Service which was undertaken in the 1980s, was that of de-hospitalisation. The placing of care in the community, gathered momentum and by the 1990s, some of the famous teaching hospitals which represented the traditional power base of the medical profession were being closed down. This move was reflected in the plans for the reorganisation of childbirth with the proposal to place more care in midwifery-led units and to offer more home births.

But how can we 'understand' this move towards a managerial rather than a professional-based power structure? The professions represented a system of alternative power bases and as such could stand in the way of state policies. Recent governments have consistently striven to limit and control the power of professionals, not only doctors and health-care professionals but also teachers, social workers and even lawyers. The professions could be regarded as the last ethical defence against state control or they could be seen as a 'conspiracy' against democracy. The introduction of managerial control and of 'skill-mix' can be defined as a strategy to undermine and control professionalism.

■ Questions and discussion points

- Using the 'trait' approach (Millerson, 1964), decide if midwifery can be defined as a profession. Justify your answer.
- Using Witz (1992) model of strategies of control answer these questions:
  Are midwives controlled by and therefore a subordinate group to nurses?
  What is the evidence of this control?
  Is there any evidence of dual closure?
  Have midwives as a subordinate group used inclusionary tactics in accepting a separate pay structure and local pay bargaining?
- What is midwifery theory? (See Bryar 1995.) How well is theory understood and used by midwives in clinical midwifery practice?
- List the advantages and disadvantages of midwifery becoming an academic discipline.
- Is midwifery all, some or none of the following? A craft, a skill, a profession?
- Has midwifery been de-skilled or re-skilled as a result of the medicalis-ation of birth?
- Is professional regulation in the public interest?
- How do the statutory bodies protect the public?
- Does statutory supervision of midwifery demonstrate that midwifery is not a profession?
- In your area are midwives in senior managerial positions in the new health service? Consider the implications of their presence or their absence.

Key points

- The professions have been defined using a 'trait' approach, i.e. listing various characteristics as a checklist.
- Other views suggest professions are a means of control, or are a product of capitalism or a gender issue.
- Anne Witz has argued that 'because women are not men, the semi-professions are not professions'.
- Witz also argued that four main strategies are employed by occupational groups to achieve power and control. Dominant groups exercise exclusion and demarcation. Subordinate groups resist using inclusionary tactics and dual closure.
- The occupation of a female group or females within a male occupational group is termed a 'female professional project'. Midwifery can be described as a female professional project.
- Some areas of medicine have higher status than others. Gynaecology as a medical discipline has taken many years to achieve social respectability.
- It is the possession of theory or a theoretical basis for action which is an essential ingredient for professionalisation.
- There are still many individuals and groups who would wish to de-professionalise midwifery. Some are openly hostile and against the establishing of midwifery education in higher education.
- Skill is a gender-based concept.
- Midwives argue that their skills have been under-used and devalued by the medicalisation of birth. Some will argue that to claim to possess a specialised skill is not the mark of a profession but a craft. Midwives may gain greater respect and status in respect of their craft than for their professionalism.
- Midwifery may have been deskilled or reskilled as a result of the medicalisation of childbirth.
- In their struggle for professional status midwives have been in conflict with doctors and with nurses.
- Professional regulation may be more about protecting the professions' self-interest than protecting the public.
- The preparation of midwives is no longer training, it is an educational process that takes place in institutions of higher education.
- The public image of midwifery remains confused and uncertain.
- *Changing Childbirth* and other policies aimed at implementing continuity of care and making greater use of midwives' skills are difficult to implement.
- Managerialism is a new power structure set to undermine and control professionalism.

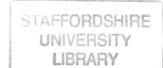

Conclusion

This book has concentrated on two major concepts in sociology: culture and power. We began by looking at the way in which power has been analysed in sociological thought and at the way cultures are constructed. We hope to have illustrated that both play a major part in the way in which women both as mothers and as midwives are perceived by society.

We next looked at social policies and their impact on women and families. It is important to remember that social policies do not 'just happen', they are the product of social structures and processes. Social policies have had a significant effect on the lives of everyone and especially upon women. To an extent the framing of policies is structured by both cultures and power structures.

When looking at the effect of policies on the working practice of midwives we have concentrated very much upon the concept of professionalisation but it is important to remember that other power structures are now in existence which threaten the whole structure and culture of professions.

The original meaning of midwife was 'with woman' and we hope that this book will play a part in enabling this supportive relationship to be improved by a wider knowledge and analysis of the social world which both now inhabit.

References

Abbott, P. and Wallace, C. (1992) *The Family and the New Right* (London: Pluto).

Ahmad, B. (1989) 'Child Care and Ethnic Minorities' in B. Kahan (ed.) (1989) *Child Care Research, Policy and Practice* (London: Hodder & Stoughton).

Allen, N. (1991) *Making Sense of the Children Act* (London: Longman).

Althusser, L. (1970) 'Ideology and Ideological State Apparatuses', *Lenin and Philosophy and Other Essays* (London: New Left Books).

Amin, K., Oppenheim, C. (1992) *Poverty in Black and White: deprivation and ethnic minorities* (CPAG and Runnymede Trust).

Andrews, A. and Jewson, N. (1993) 'Ethnicity and Infant Deaths: the implications of recent statistical evidence for materialist explanations' *Sociology of Health and Illness*, 15,2, 137–56.

Arney, W.R. (1982) *Power and the Profession of Obstetrics* (Chicago: The University of Chicago Press).

Association for Improvements in Maternity Services (1993) 'Ultrasound??? Unsound'. A special edition of the *AIMS Journal* 5 (1) 3 – 26

Association of Radical Midwives (1986) *The Vision: Proposals for the future of the maternity services* (Ormskirk, Lancashire: The Association of Radical Midwives).

Attfield, J. (1989) 'Inside Pram Town', in J. Attfield and P. Kirkham (eds) *A View From the Interior*, (London: The Women's Press).

Baggott, R. (1994) *Health and Health Care in Britain* (London: Macmillan).

Ball, J A. (1994) *Reactions to Motherhood: The Role of Post-Natal Care* (Books for Midwives Press, England).

Barker, D. (995) 'Fetal origins of coronary heart disease' *British Medical Journal* 311, 171–174.

Barnes, B. and Shapin, S. (1977) 'Science, Nature and Control: Interpreting Mechanics Institutes' *Social Studies of Science* 7, 31–74.

Barrett, M. and McIntosh, M. (1982) *The Anti-Social Family* (London: Verso).

Barrow, J. (1982) 'West Indian families: an insider's perspective' in R.Rappoport *et al.*, *Families in Britain* (London: Routledge & Kegan Paul).

Becker, H. (1973) *Outsiders: Studies in the Sociology of Deviance* (New York: Free Press).

Becker, H. (1977) *Boys in White: Student Culture in Medical School* (New Brunswick: Transaction Books).

Bedford, V. A and Johnson, N. (1988) 'The Role of the Father' *Midwifery*, Vol. 4, No 4, Dec: (1988), pp. 190–5.

Beechey, V. (1985) 'Familial Ideology', in V. Beechey and J. Donald (eds) *Subjectivity and Social Relations* (Milton Keynes: Open University).

Bell, C. and Newby, H. (1971) *Community Studies* (London: Allen & Unwin).

Bell, D. (1960) *End of Ideology* (New York: Glencoe Free Press).

Ben-David, J. (1964) 'Professions in the Class System of Present-day Societies' *Current Sociology*.

Berger, B. and Berger, P. (1983) *The War Over the Family* (London: Hutchinson).

Berger, P. and B. (1976) *Sociology: A Biographical Approach* (Harmondsworth: Penguin Education Books).

Bernstein, B. (1977) *Class Codes and Control* (London: Routledge & Kegan Paul).

Berridge, D. and Cleaver, H. (1987) *Foster Home Breakdown* (Oxford: Blackwell).

Beveridge, B. (1942) *Social Insurance and Allied Services* (London: HMSO, Cmnd. 6404).

Bhachu, P. (1985) *Twice Migrants: East African Settlers in Britain* (London: Tavistock).

Bhat, A., Carr-Hill, R., Ohri S. (1988) *Britain's Black Population: A New Perspective*, (Aldershot: Gower, Radical Statistics Race Group, 2nd edn).

Black, D., Morris, J. N., Smith, C. and Townsend, P. (1988) *The Black Report: Inequalities in Health* (Harmondsworth: Penguin).

Blackburn, C. (1991) *Poverty and Health* (Milton Keynes: Open University Press).

Blake, C. (1990) *The Charge of the Parasols: Women's Entry to the Medical Profession* (London: Women's Press).

Blakemore, K. and Boneham, M. (1993) *Age and Ethnicity* (Milton Keynes: Open University Press).

Blauner, R. (1964) *Alienation and Freedom* (Chicago: University of Chicago Press).

Bott, E. (1957) *Family and Social Networks* (London: Tavistock).

Bourke, J. (1994) *Working-Class Cultures in Britain 1890–1960* (London: Routledge).

Bowlby, J. (1953a) *Childcare and the Growth of Love* (Harmondsworth: Penguin).

Bowlby, J. (1953b) *Maternal Care and Mental Health Report* (Geneva: World Health Organisation).

Bowlby, J. (1969) *Attachment and Loss* (London: Hogarth Press).

Bowler, I. (1993) '"They're not the same as us": midwives' stereotypes of South Asian descent patients' *Sociology of Health and Illness*, 15,2, 158–177.

Bowler, I. M. W. (1993) 'Stereotypes of Women of Asian Descent in Midwifery: some evidence' *Midwifery*, 9, 7–16.

Bradshaw, J. and Millar, J. (1991) *Lone Parents in UK* (London: HMSO).

Brannen, J. (1992) 'Money, Marriage and Motherhood: Dual-earner Households after Maternity Leave' in S. Arber and N. Gilbert (eds) *Women and Working Lives; Divisions and Change* (London: Macmillan).

Brannen. J. and Moss, P. (1987) 'Fathers and employment' in C. Lewis and M. O'Brien (eds) *Reassessing Fatherhood: New Observations on Fathers and the Modern Family* (London: Sage).

Braverman, H. (1974) 'Labour and Monopoly Capital' *New York Monthly Review Press.*

Brooke, O. G., Anderson, H. R., Bland, J. M. and others (1989) 'Effects on birth weight of smoking, alcohol, caffeine, socio-economic factors and psychosocial stress' *British Medical Journal*, vol. 298, no. 66–76, 25 March 1989, pp. 795–801.

Brookes, B. (1988) *Abortion in England 1900–1967* (London: Croom Helm).

Brophy, J. (1989) 'Custody Law, Child-care and Inequality in Britain' in Smart and Sevenhuijsen (eds) *Child Custody and the Politics of Gender* (London: Routledge).

Brown, C. (1988) quoted in A. Bhatt (ed.) *Britain's Black Population: a new perspective* (Gower: Radical Statistics Race Group).

Brown, G. and Harris, T. (1978) *The Social Origins of Depression* (London: Tavistock).

Bryar, R. M. (1995) *Theory for Midwifery Practice* (London: Macmillan).

Bryson, A. and Jacobs, J. (1992) *Policing the Workshy* (Aldershot: Avebury).

Busfield, J. (1982) 'Gender and Mental Illness' *International Journal of Mental Health*, 1, 1–2, 46–66.

Butler, N. and Alberman, E. (1969) *Perinatal Problems: the second report of the 1958 British Perinatal Mortality Survey* (Edinburgh: Livingstone).

Bytheway, B. (1995) *Ageism* (Milton Keynes: Open University Press).

Campbell, B. (1993) *Goliath: Britain's Dangerous Places* (London: Methuen) p. 18.

Campbell, J. and Macfarlane, A.(1995) *Where to be Born: The Debate and the Evidence* (John Radcliffe, Oxford: National Perinatal Epidemiology Unit).

Cardwell, D. (1957) *The Organisation of Science in England* (London: Heinemann).

Carter, M. (1966) *Into Work* (Harmondsworth: Penguin).

Castles, S. and Kosack, G. (1973) *Immigrant Workers and the Class Structure* (London: Oxford University Press for Institute of Race Relations).

Chadwick, J. (1994) 'Perinatal Mortality and Antenatal Care' *Modern Midwife*, vol. 4, no. 9, September 1994, pp. 18–20.

Chalmers, I, Oakley, A. and Macfarlane, A. (1980) 'Perinatal health services: an immodest proposal' *British Medical Journal*, vol.280, no. 6217, pp. 842–5.

Chamberlain, M. (1981) *Old Wives Tales* (London: Virago).

Channel Four (1995) *War Cries Documentary*, 17 August.

Charles, N. and Kerr, C. (1988) *Women, Food and Families* (Manchester: Manchester University Press).

Chertok, L. (1969) *Motherhood and Personality* (London: Tavistock).

Chesler, P. (1972) *Women and Madness* (New York: Doubleday).

Chesler, P. (1990) *Sacred Bond: Legacy of Baby M* (London: Virago).

Chodorow, N. (1994) 'Gender Relation and Difference in Psychoanalytic Perspective' *Policy Reader in Gender Studies* (London: Policy Press).

Clark, J. (ed.) (1993) *Crisis in Care? Challenges to Social Work* (London: Sage).

Clement, S. (1995) 'Listening visits in pregnancy: a strategy for preventing post-natal depression?' *Midwifery* 11, no. 2, June, 75–80.

Cochrane, A. (1993) 'Challenges from the Centre' in C. Clarke (ed.) *A Crisis in Care? Challenges to Social Work Open University* (London: Sage).

Cockburn, C. (1985) *Machinery of Dominance: Men, Women and Technical 'Know How'* (London: Pluto Press).

Cockburn, C. (1990) *Brothers: Male Dominance and Technological Change* (London: Pluto Press).

Cockburn, C. (1993) *Gender and Technology in the Making* (London: Sage).

Cohen, S. and Taylor, L. (1992) *Escape Attempts: The Theory and Practice of Resistance to Everyday Life* (London: Routledge) 2nd edn.

Colwill, J. (1994) 'Beveridge, Women and the Welfare State' *Critical Social Policy*, 41, 14, 2, 53–78.

Cooper, D.(1972) *The Death of the Family* (Harmondsworth: Penguin).

Corden, A. and Craig, P. (1991) *Perception of Family Credit*, Social Policy Research Unit (London: HMSO).

Coward, R. (1984) 'The Royals' in V. Beechey and J. Donald (eds) *Subjectivity and Social Relations* (Milton Keynes: Open University Press).

Cox, J. L. (1986) *Post-natal Depression* (Edinburgh: Churchill Livingstone).

Cox, J. L., Murray, D., Chapman, G. (1993) 'A controlled study of the onset, duration and prevalence of post-natal depression' *British Journal of Psychiatry*, 163, pp. 27–31.

Craig, G. and Glendinning, C. (1990) *Missing the Target* (Ilford: Barnardos).

Crawford, M. A. (1993) 'The role of fatty acids in neural development: implications for perinatal nutrition' *American Journal of Clinical Nutrition 8*, 45–55

CRE [Council for Racial Equality] (1988) *Report of a Formal Investigation into St. Georges Hospital Medical School* (London: CRE).

Crompton, R. and Sanderson K. (1990) *Gendered Jobs and Social Change* (London: Unwin Hyman).

Crowther, M. (1981) *The Workhouse System 1834-1929* (London: Batsford Academic and Educational).

Crowther, M. (1982) 'Family Responsibility and State Responsibility in Britain before the Welfare State' *Historical Journal*, 25,1.

Daily Telegraph (1989) 'Midwife wins appeal over "misconduct"' 25 February 1989, p. 4.

Dale, J. and Foster, P. (1986) *Feminists and State Welfare* (London: Routledge & Kegan Paul).

Dalley, G. (1988) *Ideologies of Caring: Rethinking Community and Collectivism,* (London: Macmillan).

Dalton, K. (1980) *Depression after Childbirth* (London: Oxford University Press).

David, M. (1989)'Putting on an Act for Children?' in Stainton Rogers, Hevey, Ash (eds) *Child Abuse and Neglect* (Milton Keynes Open University).

Davidoff, L. and Hall, C. (1987) *Family Fortunes: men and women of the English middle class 1780–1850* (London: Hutchinson).

Davies, J. and Evans, F. (1991) 'The Newcastle Community Midwifery Care Project' in S. Robinson, and A. M. Thomson (eds), *Midwives, Research and Childbirth* (London: Chapman & Hall) vol. II.

Davin, A. (1978) 'Imperialism and Motherhood' *History Workshop Journal,* 5, 9–65.

Davis, R. and Moore, W (1945) 'Some principles of stratification' *American Sociological Review,* x, 2, 242–249.

de Beauvoir, S. (1972) *The Second Sex* (Harmondsworth: Penguin).

Deem, R. (1978) *Women and Schooling* (London: Routledge & Kegan Paul).

Delamont, S. (1980) *Sociology of Women* (London: George Allen & Unwin).

Delphy, C. (1977) *The Main Enemy* (London: Writers & Readers Group).

Delphy, C. (1984) *Close to Home: A Materialist Analysis of Women's Oppression,* (London: Hutchinson).

Dennis, N. and Erdos G. (1993) *Families without Fatherhood* (London: Institute of Economic Affairs Health and Welfare Unit) 2nd edn.

Dennis, N., Henriques, F. and Slaughter, C. (1969) *Coal is our Life* (London: Tavistock).

Department of Health (1991) *The Health of the Nation* (London: HMSO).

Department of Health (1993), *Changing Childbirth: Part 1–The Report of the Expert Maternity Group* (London: HMSO).

Department of Social Security (1994) *Households Below Average Income 1979–91/2: A Statistical Analysis* (London: Government Statistical Service HMSO).

Dex, S. (1987) *Women's Occupational Mobility: A Lifetime Perspective* (London: Macmillan).

Dex, S. and Shaw, L. (1986) *British and American Women at Work* (London: Macmillan).

Dick Read, G. (1951) *Childbirth without Fear* (London: Heinemann).

Dick Read, G. (1950) *Introduction to Motherhood* (London: Heinemann).

Dingwall, R. and Lewis, P. (1983) *The Sociology of the Professions* (London: Macmillan).

Dingwall, R., Rafferty, A., and Webster, C. (1988) *An Introduction to the Social History of Nursing* (London: Routledge).

Donnison, J. (1988) *Midwives and Medical Men. A History of the Struggle for the Control of Childbirth* (London: Historical Publications) 2nd edn.

Donovan, J. (1986) *We Don't Buy Sickness – It Just Comes* (Aldershot: Gower).

Donzelot, J. (1970) *Policing of Families,* 1st edn (London: Macmillan).

Donzelot, J. (1980) *The Policing of Families* (London: Hutchinson).

Dowswell, T. and Hewison, J. (1994) 'Ultrasound Examinations in Pregnancy: Some Suggestions for Debate' *Midwifery* 1994, vol. 10, no.4, pp. 181–250

Durkheim, E. (1964) *Division of Labour in Society* (London: Collier-Macmillan).

Durward, L., Evans, R. (1990) 'Pressure Groups and Maternity Care' in J. Garcia, R. Kilpatrick, and M. Richards, *The Politics of Maternity Care* (Oxford: Clarendon Paperback).

Ehrenreich, B. and English, D. (1973) *For Her Own Good: 150 years of expert advice to women* (London: Writers and Readers Cooperative).

Engels, F. (1978) *The Origin of the Family, Private Property and the State* (London: Lawrence & Wishart).

English, B. and Ehrenreich, D. (1976) *Complaints and Disorders: The Sexual Politics of Sickness* (London: Writers and Readers Publishing Cooperative).

Enkin, M, Keirse, M. J. N. C., Renfrew, M, and Nelson, J. (1995) *A Guide to Effective Care in Pregnancy and Childbirth* (Oxford: Oxford University Press) 2nd edn.

Ermisch, J. (1991) *Fewer Babies Longer Lives* (York: Joseph Rowntree Foundation) p. 15. quoted in Greve, J. *Homelessness in Britain* (Joseph Rowntree Foundation, 1991).

Essam, P. and Berthoud, R. (1991) *Independent Benefits for Men and Women* (London: Policy Studies Institute).

Etzioni, A. (1969) *The Semi-Professions and Their Organisation* (New York: Free Press).

Eyer, D. E. (1993) *Mother–Infant Bonding: A Scientific Fiction* (New Haven, Connecticut: Yale University Press).

Family Policies Study Centre (1990) *One-Parent Families* (London: Family Policies Study Centre)

Family Policy Bulletin (1991) (London: Family Policy Studies Centre) December.

Finch, J. (1984) 'The Deceit of Self-Help: Pre-School Playgroups and Working-Class Mothers', *Journal of Social Policy*, 13, 1, pp. 1–20

Finch, J. and Groves, D. (1983) *Labour of Love: Women, Work and Caring* (London: Routledge & Kegan Paul).

Firestone, S. (1970) *The Dialectic of Sex* (New York: William Morrow).

Fletcher, R. (1962) *Britain in the Sixties: the family and marriage* (Harmondsworth: Penguin).

Flint, C. (1994) *Midwifery Teams and Caseloads* (Oxford: Butterworth Heinemann).

Forrest, R. and Murie, A. (1988) *Selling the Welfare State: The Privatisation of Public Housing* (London: Routledge).

Foster, P. (1995) *Women and the Health Care Industry: an unhealthy relationship?* (Milto Keynes: Open University Press).

Foucault, M. (1973) *Birth of the Clinic* (London: Allen Lane).

Foucault, M. (1977) *Discipline and Punishment* (Harmondsworth: Penguin).

Foucault, M. (1980a) *Power/Knowledge: Selected Interviews and Other Writings* (Brighton: Harvester Press).

Foucault, M. (1980b) *Truth, Power and Sexuality* (Brighton: Harvester Press).

Frankenburg, R. (1965) *Communities* (Harmondsworth: Penguin).

Franklin, S. (1990) 'De-Constructing "Desperateness": The Social Construction of Infertility in Popular Representations of New Reproductive Technologies' in M. McNeil *et al.* (eds) *The New Reproductive Technologies* (Basingstoke: Macmillan).

Friedan, B. (1963) *The Feminine Mystique* (Harmondsworth: Penguin)

Furness, M. (1987) 'Reporting Obstetric Ultra-Sound' *Lancet*, i, 675.

Gabriel, J.,and Tovim, G. Ben (1978) 'Marxism and the concept of racism' *Economy and Society*, 7, 2.

Gans, H. (1967) 'Urbanism and suburbanism as a way of life' in R. Bocock, P. Hamilton K. Thomson and A. Watson (eds) *Introduction to Sociology* (London: Fontana).

Gavron, H. (1966) *The Captive Wife* (Harmondsworth: Penguin).

Giddens, A. (1971) *Capitalism and Modern Social Theory: An Analysis of the Writings of Marx, Durkheim and Weber* (Cambridge: Cambridge University Press).

Gillis, J. (1985) *For Better For Worse: British Marriages 1600 to the present* (London: Heinemann).

Gilroy, P. (1987), *There Ain't No Black in the Union Jack* (London: Hutchinson).

Gittins, D. (1985) *The Family in Question* (London: Macmillan).

Gluckman, M. (1990) *Women Assemble* (London: Routledge).

Goffman, E. (1961a) *Asylums* (Harmondsworth: Penguin).

Goffman, E. (1961b) *Encounters: Two Studies in the Sociology of Interaction* (Indianapolis: Bobbs-Marrill).

Goldthorpe, D. and Lockwood, D. (1968) *Affluent Worker: Industrial Attitudes and Behaviour* (Cambridge: Cambridge University Press).

Gove, W. (1984) 'Gender Differences in Mental and physical illness: The Effects of Fixed Roles and Nurturant roles' *Social Science and Medicine*, 19, 2, 77–91.

Graham, H. (1987) 'Being Poor: Perceptions and Coping Strategies of Lone Mothers' in Brannen, J. and Wilson, G. (eds) *Give and Take in Families* (London: Allen & Unwin).

Gramsci, A. (1971) *Selections from the Prison Notebooks* (London: Lawrence & Wishart).

Granshaw, H. and Porter, R. (eds) (1990) *The Hospital in History* (London: Routledge).

Green, J., Stalham, H. (1993) 'Testing for fetal abnormality in routine antenatal care' *Midwifery* 9, No.3, 124–35.

Greer, G. (1985) *Sex and Destiny: Politics of Human Fertility* (London: Secker Warburg).

Greve, J. (1991) *Homelessness in Britain* (York: Joseph Rowntree Foundation).

Guru, S. (1986) 'An Asian Women's Refuge' in S. Ahmad, J. Cheetham and J. Small, (eds) *Social Work with Black Children and Their Families* (London: Batsford).

Hakim, C. (1979) 'Occupational Segregation: A Comparative Study of the Degree and Pattern of the Differentiation Between Men and Women's Work in Britain, USA and other countries' (London: Department of Employment Research Paper).

Hall, S. and Jefferson, T. (1975) *Resistance through Rituals* (London: Hutchinson).

Hamilton (1988) *Review of Food Patterns Amongst Lower Income Groups in the UK*, a Report to Health Education Authority (unpublished).

Harkness, S., Machin, S., Waldfogel, J. (1994) 'Women's Pay and Family Income Inequality' Findings, Social Policy Research (York: Joseph Rowntree Foundation).

Harris, O. (1981) 'Households as Natural Units' in K. Young, C. Wolkowitz and R. McCullagh (eds), *Of Marriage and the Market: Women's Subordination in an International perspective* (London: Collective Socialist Economists).

Harrison, S. and Pollitt, C. (1994) *Controlling Health Professionals* (Milton Keynes: Open University Press).

Health Committee (1992) Second Report, *Maternity Services*, Vol 1, (HMSO).

Hearn, J. (1987) *The Gender of Oppression* (Brighton: Wheatsheaf).

Hearn, J. (1992) *Men in the Public Eye* (London: Routledge).

Hillery, G. (1955) 'Definitions of Community: areas of agreement' *Rural Sociology*, 20, 2, 111–23.

HMSO (1991) *Patterns and Outcomes in Child Placement* (London: HMSO).

HMSO (1995) *Social Focus on Women* (London: HMSO).

Hoggart, R.(1955) *The Uses of Literacy* (Harmondsworth: Penguin).

Holterman, S. and Clarke, R. (1992) *Parents, Employment Rights and Childcare* (London: Equal Opportunities Commission Research) Series 4.

Home Office (1995) *Domestic Violence Factsheet* (London: Home Office).

Honigsbaum, F. (1979) *The Division in British Medicine: A History of the Separation of General Practice from Hospital Care 1911–1968* (London: Kogan Page).

House of Commons Employment Committee (March 1995) *Mothers in Employment* London: HMSO).

House of Commons Health Committee (1992) *Maternity Services* (Chairman: Mr N. Winterton) (London: HMSO) vol. 1.

House of Commons Social Services Committee 1979–80 (Chairwoman: R. Short) (London: HMSO).

House of Commons, Social Services Committee (1984) *Perinatal and Neonatal Mortality Report from the Social Services Committee 1983–84* (Chairwoman: R. Short) (London: HMSO).

Hubbard, R. (1985) 'Prenatal Diagnosis and Eugenic Ideology' *Women's Studies International Forum*, 8, 6, 567–76.

Humphries J. (1977) 'Class Struggle and the Persistence of the Working-class Family' *Cambridge Journal of Economics*, 1, 1, 241–58.

Humphries, P. and Gordon, P. (1993) *Labour of Love: The Experiences of Parenthood in Britain 1900–50* (London: Sidgwick & Jackson).

Hunt, S. C. (1993a) 'The Pursuit of Scholarship' *British Journal of Midwifery*, September 1993, vol. 1, no.4, pp. 177–86.

Hunt, S. C. (1993b) 'Now is not the right time for a new Midwives Act?' *British Journal of Midwifery*, Nov./Dec. 1993, vol. 1, no. 6.

Hunt, S. C. (1995a) 'The Social Meaning of Midwifery: The Dame Rosalind Paget Memorial Lecture' *Midwives*, vol. 108, no. 1292, pp. 283–87.

Hunt, S. C. (1995b) 'A New Midwives Act. Who will really benefit?' *Modern Midwife*, Sept. 1995, pp. 30–1.

Hunt, S. C. and Symonds, A. (1995) *The Social Meaning of Midwifery* (London: Macmillan).

Illich I. (1976) *Medical Nemesis: The Expropriation of Health* (London: Pantheon Books).

Inch, S. (1989) *Birth Rights* (London: Green Print) 2nd edn.

Jackson, K. (1993) 'Time for a New Act?' *British Journal of Midwifery*, Sept.1993, vol. 1, no. 4.

Jackson, S. (1993) 'Women and the Family' in D. Richardson and V. Robinson (eds) *Introducing Women's Studies* (London: Macmillan).

Jarman, B. (1983) 'Identification of Underprivileged Areas' *British Medical Journal*, 286, 1705–09.

Jarman, B. (1984) 'Underprivileged Areas Validation and Distribution of Scores', *British Medical Journal*, 289, 1587–92.

Jearn, J. (1992) *Men in the Public Eye* (London: Routledge).

Jenkins, R. (1995) *The Law and the Midwife* (Oxford: Blackwell).

Johnson, T. (1972) *Professions and Power* (London: Macmillan).

Jones, R. (1986) *Emile Durkheim: And Introduction to Four Major Works* (London: Sage).

Joshi, H. (1984) 'Women's Participation in Paid Work: Further Analysis of Women's Employment Survey', Department of Employment Research paper 45, in G. Chamberlain and P. Gunn (eds), *Birthplace* (Chichester: Wiley).

Kahan, B. (ed.) (1989) *Child Care Research, Policy and Practice* (London: Hodder & Stoughton).

Kalra, S. (1993) 'Destruction of female fetuses: The new pandemic. Women's International Public Health Network' Reprinted in MIDIRS, *Midwifery Digest* (June 1995) 5.2., pp. 141–42.

Kennedy, I. (1973) *The Unmasking of Medicine* (London: BBC Publications).

Kennedy, J. (1992) *Eve was Framed: Women and British Justice* (London: Chatto & Windus).

Kerr, C. *et al.* (1973) *Industrialisation and Industrial Man* (Harmondsworth: Penguin).

Kiernan, K. (1992) 'The Impact of Family Disruption in Childhood on Transitions Made in Young Adult Life' *Population Studies*, vol.46.

Kitzinger, S. (1978) *Women as Mothers* (London: Fontana).

Kitzinger, S. (1980a) *The Experience of Childbirth* (Harmondsworth: Penguin) 4th edn, pp. 290.

Kitzinger, S. (1980b) *Pregnancy and Childbirth* (London: Michael Joseph):

Kitzinger, S. (1990) *The Crying Baby* (Harmondsworth: Penguin).

Kitzinger, S. (1992) 'Birth and violence against women generating hypotheses from women's accounts of unhappiness after birth', in H. Roberts (ed.) *Women's Health Matters* (London: Routledge).

Klaus, M. H. and Kennell, J. H. (1976) *Maternal Infant Bonding* (St Louis: Mosby).

La Rossa, R. and La Rossa, M. (1981) *Transition to Parenthood: How Children Change Families* (Beverly Hills: Sage).

Laing, R. D. (1971), *The Politics of the Family and Other Essays* (London: Tavistock).

Land, H. (1986) *Women and Economic Dependency* (London: Equal Opportunities Commission).

Langan, M. (1993) 'New Directions in Social Work' in C. Clarke (ed.) *Crisis in Care? Challenges to Social Work* (London: Sage).

Laslett, P. (1972) *Household and Family in Past Time* (London: Cambridge University Press).

Law, C. M., Barker, D. J. P., Richardson, W. *et al.* (1993) 'Thinness at birth in a northern industrial town' *Journal of Epidemiology and Community Health* 47, 255–9.

Leach, P. (1984) *Baby and Child* (Harmondsworth: Penguin).

Leap, N. and Hunter, B. (1993) *The Midwife's Tale* (London: Scarlett Press).

Lees, S. (1986) *Losing Out: Adolescent Girls and Sexuality* (London: Hutchinson).

Lewis, O. (1964) *The Children of Sanchez* (Harmondsworth: Penguin).

Lewis, J. (1980) *The Politics of Motherhood* (London: Croom Helm).

Lewis, C. (1986) *Becoming a Father* (Milton Keynes: Open University Press).

Liptak, G. S., Keller, B. B., Feldman, A. W. and Chamberlain, R. W. (1983) 'Enhancing Infant Development and Parent–Practitioner Interaction with the Brazelton Neonatal Assessment Scale' *Paediatrics* 72, 71–8.

Lister, R. (1991) 'Women, Economic Dependency and Citizenship' *Journal of Social Policy*, 19, 4, 445–67.

Lister, R. (1992) *Women's Economic Dependency and Social Security* (London: Equal Opportunities Commission).

Lockwood, D. (1989) *Black-Coated Worker* (Oxford: Clarendon) 2nd edn.

Lovell, T. (1980) *Pictures of Reality* (London: British Film Institute).

Lowry, S. (1992) 'Student selection' *British Medical Journal*, 305, 1352–4

Lowry, S. and MacPherson, G. (1988) 'A blot on the profession' *British Medical Journal*, 296, 657–8.

Luckhaus, L. and Dickens, L. (1991) 'Social Protection of Atypical Workers in the UK', Report for European Commission.

Lynch, M. A., Roberts, J. (1977) 'Predicting child abuse: signs of bonding failure in the maternity hospital', *British Medical Journal* 1: 624–26.

MacFarlane J. A. (1984) 'Facts, Beliefs and Misconceptions about the Bonding Process', in L. Sander and G. Chamberlain (eds) *Pregnancy Care for the 1980s*, (London: Macmillan in association with Royal Society of Medicine).

Macfarlane, A., Mugford, M., Johnson, A., Garcia, J. (1995) *Counting the Changes in Childbirth: Trends and Gaps in National Statistics* (Oxford: NPEU Radcliffe Infirmary).

Mack, J. and Lansley, S. (1985) *Poor Britain* (London: Allen & Unwin).

MacLaren, A. (1978) *Birth Control in Nineteenth Century England* (London: Croom Helm).

Maclean, M. and Groves, D. (eds) (1991) *Women's Issues in Social Policy* (London: Routledge).

MacLennan, A. H. (1978) 'An audit of obstetric practice in the management of labour' *Australian and New Zealand Journal of Obstetrics and Gynaecology* 18, 1978, p. 244, in Inch, S. *Birth Rights* (London: Green Print) 2nd edn.

MacManus, I., Maitis, S., Richards, P. (1990) 'Identification of medical school applicants from ethnic minorities' *Studies in Higher Education* 15, 57–73.

Mama, A. (1989), 'Shunned and shunted around: black women's experience of statutory agencies', in *The Hidden Struggle* (London: Race and Housing Research Unit, Runnymede Trust).

Marshall, T. H. (1963) 'Citizenship and Social Class', in *Sociology at the Crossroads* (London: Heinemann).

Mann, K. (1992) *The Making of an English Underclass* (London: Routledge & Kegan Paul).

Martin, E. (1989) *The Woman in the Body* (Milton Keynes: Open University Press).

Martyn, C. N. (1994), Fetal and infant origins of cardiovascular disease *Midwifery*, 10, 61–6

Marx, K. and Engels, F. (1970) *The German Ideology* (London: Lawrence & Wishart).

Mason, D. (1995) *Race and Ethnicity in Modern Britain* (Oxford: Oxford University Press).

Maternity Alliance Report (1995) *Poor Expectations, Poverty and Undernourishment in Preganacy.*

McLellan, D. (1979) *Marxism After Marx* (London: Macmillan).

McNaught, A. (1988) *Race and Health Policy* (London: Croom Helm).

McNichol, J. (1980) *The Movement for Family Allowances 1918–1945: A Study in Social Policy Development* (London: Heinemann).

Mead, M. (1943) *Coming of Age in Samoa: a study of adolescence and sex in primitive societies* (Harmondsworth: Penguin).

Mead, M. (1950) *Male and Female* (Harmondsworth: Penguin).

Millar, J. (1994) 'Poor Mothers and Absent Fathers: Support for Lone parents in Comparative Perspective', paper given to Social Policy Association Conference, University of Liverpool.

Millar, J. and Glendinning, C. (eds) (1987) *Women and Poverty in Britain* (Brighton: Harvester Wheatsheaf).

Millar, J. and Whiteford, P. (1993) 'Child Support in Lone-Parent Families: Policies in Australia and the UK' *Policy and Politics*, 21, 1 59–72.

Millerson, G. (1964) *The Qualifying Associations: A Study in Professionalisation* (London:

Ministry of Health (1937) *Report on Maternal Mortality, CMD5422* (London: HMSO).

Mitchell, J. (1976) 'Women and Equality' in J. Mitchell, and A. Oakley (eds) *The Rights and Wrongs of Women* (Harmondsworth: Penguin).

Mohr, J. (1984), 'Patterns of Abortion and the Response of American Physicians 1790–1930' in Leavitt, L. (ed.), *Women and Health in America* (Wisconsin: University of Wisconsin).

Mooney, J. (1993), *The Hidden Figure: domestic violence in North London* (London: Islington Council).

Morris, L. (1990) *The Workings of the Household* (Cambridge: Policy Press).

Morris, L. (1994), *Dangerous Classes: the Underclass and Social Citizenship* (London: Routledge).

Moscucci, O. (1990) *The Science of Woman: Gynaecology and Gender in England 1800–1929* (Cambridge: Cambridge University Press).

Mothers in Employment Maternity Action No 68 April–June 1995 pp. 1–2. Reprinted in MIDIRS. *Midwifery Digest*, September 1995, 5.3 p. 361.

Mumford, C. (1945) 'On the future of London' *Architectural Review*, 97, 577, 3–10

Murray, C. (1990) *The Emerging British Underclass* (London: IEA Health and Welfare Unit).

Noble, Smith and Munby (1992) *The Take-up of Family Credit* (Oxford: Department of Applied Social Sciences and Social Research, University of Oxford).

Newman, J. (1995) 'The Limits of Management: Gender and the Politics of Change' in J. Clarke, A. Cochrane, and E. McLaughlin (eds), *Managing Social Policy* (London: Sage).

Newton, N. (1955) *Maternal Emotions* (New York: Harper & Row).

Nicolson, P. (1993) 'Motherhood and Women's Lives' Ch. 9, p. 201, in D. Richardson and V. Robinson (eds), *Introducing Women's Studies Feminist Theory and Practice* (London: Macmillan).

Nilsson, A. (1972) 'Parental Emotional Adjustment' in N. Morris (ed.) *Psychosomatic Medicine in Obstetrics and Gynaecology* (New York: Wiley).

Northern Ireland Unit Study Group (1994) *Delivering Choice.*

Northern Ireland Unit Study Group (1995) *Translating the Vision into Reality: action plan for midwives.*

Norton, L. B., Peipert, J. F., Zierler, S. *et al.* (March 1995) 'Battering in Pregnancy: An Assessment of Two Screening Methods' *Obststrics and Gynaecology* vol. 85, no. 3 pp. 321–5 p. 296.

Nurses, Midwives and Health Visitors Act, 1979 (London: HMSO).

Nurses, Midwives and Health Visitors Act, 1992 (London: HMSO).

O'Connor, M. (1995) *Birth Tides Turning towards Home Births* (London: Pandora).

O'Driscoll, K. and Meagher, D. (1986) *Active Management of Labour* (London: Bailliere Tindall) 2nd edn.

O'Driscoll, M. (1994) 'Midwives, Childbirth and Sexuality 1' *British Journal of Midwifery*, vol. 2, no. 1, pp. 39–41, and 'Midwives, Childbirth and Sexuality 2 Men and Sex' *British Journal of Midwifery*, vol. 2, no. 2, pp. 74–6.

Oakley, A. (1974b) *The Sociology of Housework* London: Martin Robinson).

Oakley, A. (1974a) *Housewife* (London: Allen Lane).

Oakley, A. (1985) *Sex Gender and Society* (London: Gower) 2nd edn.

Oakley, A. (1986) *The Captured Womb* (Oxford: Blackwell).

Oakley, A. (1989) 'Smoking in Pregnancy: Smokescreen or Risk Factor? Towards a Materialist Analysis' *Sociology of Health and Illness*, vol. 11, no. 4, pp. 311–35.

Oakley, A. (1994) 'Giving support in pregnancy: The Role of Research Midwives in a Randomised, Controlled Trial' in S. Robinson and Ann M. Thomson (eds.) *Midwives Research and Childbirth*, vol. 3, Ch.3.

Oakley, A., Rajan, L. and Grant, A. (1990) 'Social Support and Pregnancy Outcome' *British Journal of Obstetrics and Gynaecology*, no. 97, pp. 155–62.

Odent, M. (1994) 'Launching the CENEP (Campaign for Eliminating the Nocebo Effect of Prenatal Care)' *Primal Health Research – A New Era in Health Research.* vol. 2, no.2, Sept 1994, pp. 3–6 Reprinted in MIDIRS *Midwifery Digest*, March 1995, 5:1, p. 31–2

Ooscucci O. (1990) *The Science of Woman: Gynaecology and Gender in England 1800–1929* (Cambridge: Cambridge University Press).

OPCS (1994) (Office of Population Censuses and Surveys) *Social Trends*, 24.

OPCS (1995) (Office of Population Censuses and Surveys) *Monitor DH3*, 95/3 no 26. December 1995 Infant and Perinatal Mortality, Social and Biological Factors.

Ortner, S. (ed) (1981) *Sexual Meanings: The Cultural Construction of Gender and Sexuality* (Cambridge: Cambridge University Press).

Owen, D. (1992), *Ethnic Minorities in Great Britain – Settlement Patterns* (Warwick University Centre for Research in Ethnic Relations).

Owusu-Bempah, J. (1989) 'The New Institutional Racism', *Community Care*,780

Pahl, R. (1965) *Urbs in Rure* (London: Weidenfeld & Nicolson).

Pahl, J. (1989) *Money and Marriage* (London: Macmillan).

Pahl, J. (1995), 'Health Professionals and Violence against Women' in P. Kingston and B. Penhale (eds), *Family Violence and the Caring Professions* (London: Macmillan).

Parke, R. D. (1981) *Fathering Glasgow* (Fontana) cited in D. Richardson and V. Robinson (eds), *Introducing Women's Studies* (London: Macmillan).

Parkin, F. (1971) *Class Inequality and Political Order* (London: MacGibbon & Kee).

Parsons, T. (1954) *Essays in Social Theory* (London: Collier-Macmillan).

Parsons, T. (1964) 'Some Theoretical Considerations Bearing on the Field of Medical sociology' in *Social Structure and Personality* (London: Collier-Macmillan).

Peat Marwick McLintock Report (1989) Review of the United Kingdom Central Council and the Four National Board for Nursing Midwifery and Health Visiting. Commission by Department of Health, Scottish Home and Health Department, Welsh Office, Departmental of health and Social Services, Northern Ireland Crown Copyright.

Pember Reeves M. (1911) *Roundabout a Pound a Week* (London: Virago).

Penn, R., Martin, A., Scattergood, H. (1990) *Employment Trajectories of Asian Workers*, ESRC Working Paper 14.

Percival, R (1970) 'Management of Normal Labour' *The Practitioner* 1221, March, p. 204.

Petchesky, R. (1987) 'Foetal Images: The Power of Visual Culture in the Politics of Reproduction' in M. Stanworth (ed.) *Reproductive Technology* (Cambridge: Polity Press).

Pharaoh, P. O. D., Stevenson, C. J., Cooke, R. W. I. and Stevenson, R. C. (1990) 'Birth weight specific trends in cerebral palsy' *Archives of Diseases in Childhood* 65, 602–6.

Phillipson, C. (1982) *Capitalism and the Construction of Old Age* (London: Macmillan).

Pilgrim, D. and Rogers, A. (1993) *A Sociology of Mental Health and Illness* (Milton Keynes: Open University Press).

Pitt, B. (1968) 'A Typical Depression Following Childbirth' *British Journal of Psychiatry*, 114, 1325–35.

Price, F. (1990) 'The Management of Uncertainty in Obstetric Practice' in M. McNeil *et al., The New Reproductive Technologies* (London: Macmillan).

RCOG (1983) Report of the RCOG Ethics Committee on *In Vitro* Fertilisation and Embryo Replacement and Transfer (London: RCOG).

Reid, T. (1994) 'Birth Rite', *Nursing Times*, vol. 90, no.50, 14 Dec 1994, p. 16.

Rex, J. and Moore, R. (1967) *Race, Community and Conflict* (Oxford: Oxford University Press).

Rex, J. and Tomlinson, S. (1978) *Colonial Immigrants in a British City – A Class Analysis* (London: Routledge & Kegan Paul).

Richardson, D. (1993) *Women, Motherhood and Child-Rearing* (London: Macmillan).

Riley, D. (1984) *War in the Nursery* (London: Virago).

Roberts, M. (1991) *Living in a Man-made World: Gender Assumptions in Modern Housing Design* (London: Routledge).

Roberts, R. (1973) *The Classic Slum: Salford Life in the First Quarter of the Century* (Harmondsworth: Penguin).

Robinson, S. (1989) 'Caring for Child-bearing Women: The Interrelationship Between Midwifery and Medical Responsibilities', in S. Robinson and A. M. Thompson (eds), *Midwives, Research and Childbirth* (London: Chapman & Hall) vol. 1.

Roch, S. (1995) 'Midwifery Education Betrayed' *British Journal of Midwifery*, April 1995, vol. 3, no. 4, p. 186.

Roderick, G. and Stephenson, M. (1972) *Scientific and Technical Education in Nineteenth Century England* (Newton Abbot: David & Charles).

Rosser, C. and Harris, C. (1965) *The Family and Social Change* (London: Routledge & Kegan Paul).

Roth, R. (1993) 'At Women's Expense:The Costs of Fetal Rights' in Merrick, J. and Blank, R. (eds) *The Politics of Pregnancy* (New York: Harrington Park Press).

Rowbotham, S. (1973) *Hidden From History* (London: Pluto Press).

Rowe, J., Handleby, M. and Garnett, L. (1989) *Child Care Now: A Survey of Placement Patterns* (London: British Agencies for Adoption and Fostering).

Rowntree, Joseph, Foundation (1990) 'The Contribution of the Social Fund to Relieving Poverty' *Social Policy Research Findings 8.*

Rowntree, Joseph, Foundation (1991) 'The Performance of the Social Fund' *Social Policy Research Findings 14.*

Rowntree, Joseph, Foundation (1994) 'Trends in Applications for the Family Fund' *Social Policy Research Findings 53.*

Royal College of Midwives (1991) *Report of the Royal College of Midwives Commission on Legislation Relating to Midwives* (London: Royal College of Midwives).

Royal College of Midwives. (1991) *Towards a Healthy Nation. Every Day a Birth Day* (London: Royal College of Midwives).

Sandall, J. (1995) 'Burnout and Midwifery: An Occupational Hazard?' *British Journal of Midwifery*, May 1995, vol. 3, no. 5.

Schwartz-Cowan, R. (1989) *More Work For Mother: The Ironies of Household Technology from the Open Hearth to the Microwave* (London: Free Association Books).

Schwarz, E. W. (1990) 'The Engineering of Childbirth: A New Obstetric Programme as Reflected in British Obstetric Textbooks, 1960–1980' in Garcia, G., Kilpatrick, R. and Richards, M. (eds) *The Politics of Maternity Care* (Oxford: Clarendon Paperbacks) pp. 47–60.

Segal, L. (ed.) (1983) *What is to be Done about the Family?* (Harmondsworth: Penguin).

Selman, P. (1994) 'Teenage Motherhood – Then and Now: a comparison of the pattern and outcomes of teenage pregnancy in England' Association Conference on Families in Question at Liverpool University, July 1994.

Sennett, R. (1977) *The Fall of Public Man* (Cambridge: Cambridge University Press).

Sharpe, S. (1994) *Fathers and Daughters* (London: Routledge).

Shorter, E. (1977) *The Making of the Modern Family* (London: Fontana).

Silverton, L (1993) *The Art and Science of Midwifery* (London: Prentice-Hall).

Simpson, R. and Simpson, I. (1969) 'Women and Bureaucracy in the Semi-professions', in A. Etzioni (ed.) *The Semi-Professions and their Organization* (New York: Free Press).

Sloane, P. and Jain, H. (1989) *The Development of Equal Opportunity Policies in North America and Europe: An Overview* (Aberdeen: Dept of Economics, University of Aberdeen).

Smith, F. B. (1979) *The Peoples' Health, 1830–1910* (London: Croom Helm).

Smith, R. (1993) 'Academic Medicine: Plenty of Room at the Top', *British Medical Journal*, 306, 6.

Smith, R. (1993) 'Deception in Research and Racial Discrimination in Medicine' *British Medical Journal*, 306, 668–9.

Smith-Rosenberg, C. (1984) 'The Hysterical Woman: Sex Roles and Conflict in 19th Century America' in N. Black *et al.* (eds) *Health and Disease: A Reader* (Milton Keynes: Open University Press).

Smith, S. (1987) 'Residential segregation: a geography of English racism?' *Race and Racism: essays in social geography* (London: Allen & Unwin).

Spender, D. and S. (eds) (1988) *Learning to Lose: Sexism and Education* (London: Women's Press).

Spender, D. (1990) *Man-Made Language* (London: Pandora Press).

Squire, J. (1984) 'Ultra-Sound' *AIMS Quarterly*, Summer.

Stacey, M. (1960) *Tradition and Change: A Study of Banbury* (London: Oxford University Press) p. 17.

Stanworth, M. (1983) *Gender and Schooling* (London: Hutchinson).

Stanworth, M. (ed) (1987) *Reproductive Technologies: Gender, Motherhood and Medicine* (Cambridge: Polity Press).

Stock, J. and Wraight A. (1993) *Developing Continuity of Care in Maternity Services. The Implications for Midwives* (Institute of Manpower Studies, Royal College of Midwives University of Sussex).

Stone, K. (1983) 'Motherhood and Waged Work: West Indian, Asian and White Mothers Compared' in A. Phizacklea (ed.), *One-Way Ticket: Migration and Female Labour* (London: Routledge).

Stone, L. (1990) *Road to Divorce: England 1530–1987* (Oxford: Clarendon).

Stone, M. (1979) *The Paradise Papers* (London: Virago).

Stoppard, M. (1984) *The Babycare Book* (London: Dorling Kindersley).

Strong, P. and Robinson, J. (1990) *The NHS Under New Management* (Milton Keynes: Open University Press).

Summersgill, P. (1993) 'Couvade – the retaliation of marginalised fathers', ch.6 in J. Alexander, V. Levy, and S. Roch (eds), *Midwifery Practice: A Research Based Approach* (London: Macmillan).

Taylor, M. (1990) 'When enough is enough?' *Fertility and Sterility*, 54,5, 772–74.

Taylor-Gooby, P. (1990) 'Social Welfare – The Unkindest Cut of All' in R. Jowell (ed.), *British Social Attitudes: The Seventh Report, Social and Community Planning Research* (Aldershot: Gower).

Tew, M. (1995) *Safer Childbirth: A Critical History of Maternity Care* (London: Chapman Hall) 2nd edn.

Thoburn, J.(1994) *Child Placement: Principles and Practice* (Aldershot: Arena).

Tonnies, F. (1957) *Community and Society* (New York: Harper & Row).

Towler, J. and Bramall, J. (1986) *Midwives in History and Society* (London: Croom Helm).

Townsend, P. (1979) *Poverty in the UK* (Harmondsworth: Penguin).

Townsend, P., Simpson, D., Tibbs, N. (1985) 'Inequalities in Health in the City of Bristol' *International Journal of Health Services*, 15, 4, 637–63.

Townsend, P. and Davidson, N. (1982) *The Black Report* (Harmondsworth: Penguin).

United Kingdom Central Council for Nursing, Midwifery and Health Visiting *Statistical Analysis of the Council's Professional Register. April 1993–March 1994* (London: UKCC, Sept. 94).

United Kingdom Central Council for Nursing, Midwifery and Health Visiting (1993) 'The Council's Proposed standard for Post-Registration Education', Annexe 2 to Registrar's Letter 8/1993 (London: UKCC).

United Kingdom Central Council for Nursing, Midwifery and Health Visiting (1990) *The Report of the Post Registration Education and Practice Project* (London: UKCC).

United Kingdom Central Council for Nursing, Midwifery and Health Visiting *Midwives Rules, November 1993* (London: UKCC).

Ungerson, C. (1987) *Policy is Personal: Sex, Gender and Informal Care* (London: Tavistock).

Van Every, J. (1992) 'Who is "the family"? The assumptions of British social policy' *Critical Social Policy* , 33, 62–75.

Veblen, T. (1975) *Theory of the Leisure Class* (London: Unwin).

Walby, S. (1986) *Patriarchy at Work: Patriarchy and Capitalist Relations in Employment* (Cambridge: Polity).

Walby, S. (1990) *Theorizing Patriarchy* (Oxford: Blackwell).

Walby, S., Greenwell, J., Mackay, L. and Soothill, K. (1994) *Medicine and Nursing* (London: Sage).

Walker, A. (1980) 'The Social Creation of Poverty and Dependency in Old Age' *Journal of Social Policy* 9, 49–75.

Walkowitz, J. (1982a) 'Jack the Ripper and the Myth of Male Violence' *Feminist Studies*, 8, 543–74.

Walkowitz, J. (1982b) 'Male Vice and Feminist Virtue: Feminism and the Politics of Prostitution in Nineteenth-century Britain' *History Workshop Journal*, 13, 77–93.

Walkowitz, J. (1992) *City of Dreadful Delight* (London: Virago).

Wallerstein, J. and Kelly, J. (1980) *Surviving the Break-Up* (London: Grant McIntyre).

Warner, M. (1976) *Alone of All Her Sex: The Myth and Cult of the Virgin Mary* (London: Weidenfeld & Nicolson).

Warwick, C. (1995) 'Tensions in the system' *British Journal of Midwifery*, July 1995, vol. 3, no. 7, pp. 358–9.

Watson, S. and Austerberry, H. (1986) *Housing and Homelessness: A Feminist Perspective* (London: Routledge).

Weber, M. (1948) in *From Max Weber H. Gerth and C. W. Mills* (translators and editors) (London: Routledge & Kegan Paul).

Weber, M. (1930) *The Protestant Ethic and the Spirit of Capitalism* (London: Allen & Unwin).

Weeks, J. (1981) *Sex, Politics and Society* (London: Longman).

Welsh Health Planning Forum (August 1991) *Protocol for Investment in Health Gain in Maternal and Early Child Health* (Welsh Health Planning Forum).

Werbner, P. (1989) *The Migration Process* (New York: Berg).

Whitehead, M. (1988) *The Health Divide* (Harmondsworth: Penguin).

Wilkinson, R. G. (1994) 'Health redistribution and growth' in A. Glyn and D. Milibrand (eds), *Paying for Inequality: the Economic Cost of Social Injustice* (London: Oram).

Williams, P., Tarnopolosky, A., Hand, A., Shephers, M. (1986) 'Minor psychiatric morbidity and general practice consultations; the West London study' *Psychological Medicine Monograph*, Supplement 9.

Williams, J. and Watson, G. (1988) 'Sexual inequality, family life and family therapy', Street, E. and Dryden, W. (eds) *Family Therapy in Britain* (Milton Keynes: Open University Press).

Williams, F. (1989) *Social Policy* (Cambridge: Polity Press).

Williams, R. (1977) *The Country and the City* (London: Chatto & Windus).

Willis, P. (1980) *Learning to Labour: How Working-class Kids Get Working-class Jobs* (Aldershot: Gower).

Wilmot, P. and Young, M. (1960) *Family and Kinship in East London* (Harmondsworth: Penguin Books).

Wilson, E. (1977) *Women and the Welfare State* (London: Tavistock).

Wilson, E. (1989) 'In a different way' in K. Gieve (ed.), *Balancing Acts: On Being a Mother* (London: Virago).

Witherspoon, S. and Prior, G. (1991) 'Working Mothers – Free to Choose?' in R. Jowell, L. Brook and B. Taylor, (eds) *British Social Attitudes: The 8th Report* (Aldershot: SCPR).

Witz, A. (1992) *Professions and Patriarchy* (London: Routledge).

Worden, J. William (1991) *Grief Counselling and Grief Therapy* (London: Routledge) 2nd edn.

World Health Organisation (1983) *Having a Baby in Europe* (Copenhagen: WHO) Public Health in Europe, 26.

Wynn, M. (1995) 'Has There Ever Been a Better Time to Have a Baby?' *Modern Midwife*, vol.5, no.2, Feb 1995, pp. 37–8.

Young, M. (1971) *Knowledge and Control: New Dimensions in the Sociology of Education* (London: Collier-Macmillan).

Zaretsky, E. (1976) *Capitalism, the Family and Personal Life* (London: Pluto Press).

Index